A GUIDE TO PREVENTING BACK SURGERY

A Groundbreaking Approach to Conquering Back Pain

DR. MARK D. LOSAGIO DC
DAAPM, DIBCN, FIACN

Important Information For the Reader

This information presented in this book has been compiled from my clinical experience and research. It is offered as a view of the relationship between diet, exercise, emotions, and health. This book is not intended for, self diagnosis or treatment of disease, nor is it a substitute for the advice and care of a licensed health care provider. Sharing of the information in this book with the attending physician is highly desirable.

This book is intended solely to help you make better judgements concerning your long-term health goals. If you are experiencing health problems, you should consult a qualified physician immediately. Remember early examination and detection are important to successful treatment of all diseases.

TABLE OF CONTENTS

Chapter 1: The Opioid Epidemic 1

Chapter 2: Appreciating The Miracle Of Life 16

Chapter 3: What Is "Health?" 24

Chapter 4: The Health Model Vs. The Sick Model 36

Chapter 5: Phases Of Healing 48

Chapter 6: The Low Back Pain Statistics 59

Chapter 7: Spinal Degeneration 76

Chapter 8: The Dangers And Risks Of Anesthesia And Spinal Surgery 87

Chapter 9: The Dangers Of Corticosteroid Injections 94

Chapter 10: Statin Medications And Their Connection To Back Pain 107

Chapter 11: Inflammatory Syndrome - How To Counteract The Effects Of This Silent Killer 119

Chapter 12: The Destructive Effects Of Sugar 129

Chapter 13: Eat Your Way Out Of Pain The Anti-Inflammation Diet 140

Chapter 14: A Nutritional Approach To Reducing Spinal Inflammation 153

Chapter 15: The Power Of The Pro-Adjuster 169

Chapter 16: Understanding The Basics Of Decompression Therapy 179

Chapter 17: How The Accu-Spina Decompression System Can Help Your Back Pain 193

Chapter 18: The Power Of Red Light Therapy 211

Chapter 19: How The Neuromed System Can Help Your Back Pain 222

CHAPTER 1: THE OPIOID EPIDEMIC

What Is Going On With The Opioid Epidemic In The United States?

Opioids are substances that act on opioid receptors to produce morphine-like effects. Medically they are primarily used for pain relief, including anesthesia. Other medical uses include suppression of diarrhea, treating opioid use disorder, reversing opioid overdose, suppressing cough, and suppressing opioid-induced constipation.

Opioids are a type of medicine often used to help relieve pain. They work by lowering the number of pain signals your body sends to your brain. They also change how your brain responds to pain. Doctors most often prescribe opioids to relieve pain from toothaches and dental procedures, injuries, surgeries, and chronic conditions such as cancer.

Opioids usually are safe when you use them correctly. But people who do not follow their doctor's instructions and those who misuse opioids can become addicted. Abusing opiates means that you don't follow your doctor's instructions on how to take medicine. It can also mean that you take the drug illegally.

According to the National Institute for Drug Abuse (NIDA), opioids are medications that relieve pain. These drugs reduce the intensity of pain signals reaching the brain and affect those brain areas controlling emotion, which diminishes the effects of a painful stimulus. But, from a random prescribing of opioids, the threat of gross abuse also looms large on the society.

At least 44 people die every day in the United States as a result of a prescription opioid overdose, says the Center for Disease Control and Prevention (CDC). "Drug overdose was the leading cause of injury death in 2013. Among people 25 to 64 years old, drug overdose caused more deaths than motor vehicle traffic crashes," it states.

These are indeed petrifying figures. Urging doctors to curtail prescribing random opioids, the CDC says, "An increase in painkiller prescribing is a key driver of the increase in prescription overdoses." America is in the grip of an epidemic of drug abuse, and the prescription drug abuse helpline numbers are busier than ever.

Even the governments - both federal and in states - have been worried the way drug overdoses, mostly of prescription opioids, have been claiming lives across the U.S. The U.S. Government has been doing all it can to curb the epidemic of prescription drug abuse.

What Are The Specific Numbers Regarding The Number Of People Addicted To Pain Pills In The United States?

The current opioid epidemic is the deadliest drug crisis in American history. Overdoses, fueled by opioids, are the leading cause of death for Americans under 50 years old — killing roughly 64,000 people last year, more than guns or car accidents, and doing so at a pace faster than the H.I.V. epidemic did at its peak.

The opioid epidemic has been affecting millions in the country. The 2016 National Survey on Drug Use and Health (NSDUH) suggests that 11.8 million Americans aged 12 or older misused opioids in the year. The country reported highest opioid misuse among young adults aged 18 to 25, recording an annual incidence of 7.3 percent in the past year. The opioid epidemic has been claiming thousands of lives each year. According to the Centers for Disease Control and Prevention (CDC), misusing opioids - heroin, fentanyl and prescription drugs - led to 33,091 deaths in 2015. Moreover, non-fatal unintentional opioid poisoning contributed to around 53,000 hospitalizations, and 92,262 Emergency Department (ED) visits across the country.

Heroin, in particular, wreaked havoc in the past years. The CDC reported a two-time increase in heroin use among young adults aged 18 to 25 in the past decade. With the increased use of the drug, heroin-related overdose deaths have also grown significantly, witnessing a four-fold increase since 2010. Heroin-related overdose death rates saw a 20.6 percent increase between 2014 and 2015, with around 13,000 people dying from the same in 2015 alone.

How Do These Numbers Compare To Other Countries In The World?

There is a serious epidemic surfacing among teenagers today. Oxycontin has become a popular drug choice for teenagers even after reports of deaths due to overdose. Many Hollywood celebrities have confessed to being hooked on this drug and have entered rehab. Even with all the information about the dangers of misusing this prescription, many kids are still stealing it from their parent's medicine cabinets. There is no physical need for the pain pills by many people, and they are just used to alter their states of mind.

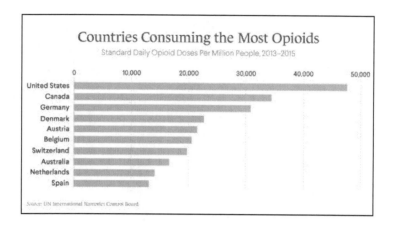

That would be on top of all the death that America has already seen in the course of the ongoing opioid epidemic. In 2016, nearly 64,000 people died of drug overdoses in America — with synthetic opioids (such as fentanyl), heroin, and common opioid painkillers (like Percocet and OxyContin) topping other causes of overdose, according to new data from the Centers for Disease Control and Prevention. That's a higher death toll than guns, car crashes, and HIV/AIDS ever killed in one year in the US, and a higher death toll than all US military casualties in the Vietnam and Iraq wars combined.

And the opioid epidemic was a key contributor to American life expectancy dropping for two years in a row in 2015 and 2016 — the first time there's been a two-year drop in US life expectancy since the early 1960s.

Are There Any Countries That Have Similar Addiction Problems Like The United States?

Drug addiction is a global problem, affecting the people of every country in the world. The ways those governments react offer a plethora of new ideas in approaching the questions of helping addicts, removing the stigma of substance abuse, and starving the black markets that exploit vulnerable people. While the efforts of the United States grab the most headlines, how other countries deal with addiction and treatment adds vital pieces to the puzzle of fighting back against drug abuse.

Although reducing the number of prescriptions will decrease the number of people who become addicted to opioids, too many prescribing restrictions could deny opioids to patients who need and benefit from them. How can we know if and when prescribing controls have gone overboard, and the population has insufficient access to prescription opioids? In short, how will we know if the effort to restrict opioids has gone too far?

United Nations data provide one important benchmark against which to judge how much more or less opioid consumption might be appropriate for a given country. And what it finds about the United States is jaw-dropping: Even when the list is restricted to the top 10 heaviest consuming countries, the United States outpaces them all in opioid use.

Here is how other countries are dealing with opioid addiction:

Amid a growing opioid crisis of its own, Canada has authorized the opening of supervised consumption sites and partnered with China to curb fentanyl flows into the country, but the health ministry says "huge gaps" remain in the government's ability to track and respond to the problem. A government report on opioid-related deaths in 2016 was the first attempt at a nationwide tally. Meanwhile, British Colombia and Alberta, two of Canada's most populous provinces, have declared a public health emergency and crisis, respectively, boosting funding for addiction treatment and increasing access to naloxone.

Also, Heroin use in Australia declined following an abrupt shortage of the drug in 2000, but the country has seen a sharp increase in the use of prescription opioids, now the cause of more than two-thirds of opioid-related deaths there. In 2012, the health ministry announced it would launch a nationwide electronic system already being used in Tasmania to monitor opioid prescriptions, but it has not yet been rolled out. The government is expected to ban over-the-counter painkillers containing codeine starting in 2018, noting that the move is a "very broad-brush approach" to the issue.

The Netherlands permits the sale and use of small amounts of cannabis to steer users away from so-called hard drugs, such as cocaine and heroin, and has implemented harm-reduction policies. In the 1990s the country began offering heroin at no cost, and the rate of high-risk or so-called problem use has halved from 2002 to some fourteen thousand in 2012, according to the European Monitoring Centre for Drugs and Drug Addiction. Proponents of decriminalization point to the Netherlands for evidence that these policies work, though critics claim they have not curbed organized crime.

How Did This Problem Start?

Over the past two decades, as the prevalence of chronic pain and health care costs have exploded, an opioid epidemic with adverse consequences has escalated. Efforts to increase opioid use and a campaign touting the alleged undertreatment of pain continue to be significant factors in the escalation. Many arguments in favor of opioids are based solely on traditions, expert opinion, practical experience and uncontrolled anecdotal observations. Over the past 20 years, the liberalization of laws governing the prescribing of opioids for the treatment of chronic non-cancer pain by the state medical boards has led to dramatic increases in opioid use.

This has evolved into the present stage, with the introduction of new pain management standards by the Joint Commission on the Accreditation of Healthcare Organizations (JCAHO) in 2000, an increased awareness of the right to pain relief, the support of various organizations supporting the use of opioids in large doses, and finally, aggressive marketing by the pharmaceutical industry.

The opioid epidemic began in the 1990s when doctors became increasingly aware of the burdens of pain. Pharmaceutical companies saw an opportunity and pushed doctors — with misleading marketing about the safety and efficacy of the drugs — to prescribe opioids to treat all sorts of pain. Doctors, many exhausted by dealing with difficult-to-treat pain patients, complied — in some states, writing enough prescriptions to fill a bottle of pills for each resident. The drugs proliferated, making America the world's leader in opioid prescriptions.

How Did Oxycontin Get Away With This Epidemic?

The sources of the opioid epidemic are complex, but one powerful motivator has been the pursuit of profit. Oxycodone is the most widely used recreational opioid in America. The U.S. Department of Health and Human Services estimates that about 11 million people in the U.S. consume oxycodone in a non-medical way annually.

Oxycodone was first made available in the United States in 1939. In the 1970s, the FDA classified oxycodone as a Schedule II drug, indicating a high potential for abuse and addiction. In 1996 Purdue Pharma introduced a new drug – a time-released formulation of oxycodone, an opioid painkiller. OyxContin, as the drug was called, was touted as having a low risk of addiction.

In 2010, Purdue Pharma reformulated OxyContin, using a polymer to make the pills extremely difficult to crush or dissolve in water to reduce OxyContin abuse. The FDA approved relabeling the reformulated version as abuse-resistant.

Purdue backed OxyContin with an aggressive marketing campaign. Key components of this effort were pain-management and speaker-training conferences in sunshine states such as California and Florida, attended by more than 5,000 physicians, nurses and pharmacists, many of whom were recruited to serve on Purdue's speakers' bureau.

The company also used a bonus system to incentivize its pharmaceutical representatives to increase OxyContin sales. The average bonus exceeded the representatives' annual salaries.

What Did The Drug Company Behind Oxycontin Tell Consumers About The Non-Addictive Properties Of The Drug?

Oxycontin is a very powerful pain reliever that is usually prescribed for people who have broken bones, severe back injuries, pain from cancer and other painful injuries or conditions. This drug is an opiate like heroin or morphine and is very addictive. If you have ever been prescribed this drug, you may have needed to have medical help with weaning yourself from it.

Opioids are drugs derived from the juice of the opium poppy, including heroin and prescription painkillers, or their synthetic equivalents, such as fentanyl. The best-known painkiller and the one attracting the most criticism for its part in America's opioid crisis is OxyContin.

For many years, doctors were wary of prescribing strong opioids, except in cases of extreme pain or palliative care, because of their well-known addictive properties. But Purdue Pharma, which was acquired by the doctors Raymond and Mortimer Sackler in the mid-20th century, sought to change this.

Their breakthrough product was a slow-release morphine pill, MS Contin. The drug dissolved gradually over several hours in a patient's bloodstream, allowing cancer patients to sleep through the night. When MS Contin's patent was due to expire, Purdue decided to develop a new drug that could be used much more widely for chronic pain. Instead of morphine, which carried a stigma among patients who weren't terminally ill, Purdue designed a new slow-release pill made of pure oxycodone, another, more powerful, chemically derived from opium.

Purdue launched OxyContin in 1996, making a bold claim: one dose relieved pain for 12 hours, twice as long as generic alternatives. The company paid doctors and funded research to support the case that the addiction risk was exaggerated and that the drug was effective for a wide range of ailments, including less severe, long-term complaints such as back pain. As the New Yorker reported in October, Purdue marketed OxyContin as a remedy to "start with and to stay with."

The pill was effective in helping many people with chronic pain who until then had received inadequate treatment and, by 2001, annual sales exceeded $1bn. But controversy was mounting. For some people, the drug only lasted for six or eight hours, resulting in withdrawal symptoms. This created "a cycle of crash and euphoria that one academic called 'a perfect recipe for addiction.'" Sales reps told doctors, many of whom mistakenly believed that oxycodone was weaker than morphine, to prescribe stronger doses rather than more frequent ones, increasing the risk of overdose. And addicts had worked out that the pills could be crushed and snorted for a quick, intense high.

Purdue settled a number of class action suits before they came to trial. But in 2007 it was charged by the US federal government with "misbranding a drug with intent to defraud or mislead." The company paid $635m in fines, one of the largest pharmaceutical settlements in US history, and three executives pleaded guilty to misdemeanor charges. But sales continued to soar.

Why Do We Have Such A Major Problem With The Opioid Pain Pill Problem?

Amid the growing opioid crisis in the United States, the capacity of available treatment programs is falling short of demand. As a result, people needing treatment for dependency on heroin or prescription painkillers have to wait for months, sometimes even years, to get appointments with certified doctors or to find slots in rehabilitation programs. While waiting to consult the experts, they are at risk of contracting HIV or hepatitis infections, as well as dying from a drug overdose.

The pain-pill epidemic has also forced doctors to consider their role. Doctors have a duty to relieve suffering, and many of us became doctors to help people. But giving that help isn't straightforward, especially when it comes to chronic pain. Try explaining the downsides of narcotics to a patient while declining to give him the medication he wants. He might accuse you of not understanding because you're not the one in pain; he might question why you won't give him what another doctor prescribed; he might give you a bad rating on a doctor-grading Web site. He might even accuse you of malpractice. None of this is rewarding for doctors: we're frustrated that we can't cure the pain and that our patients end up upset with us.

Doctors have a hard time saying no, whether a patient is asking for a narcotic to relieve pain or an antibiotic for the common cold. We are predisposed to say yes, even if we know it isn't right. Some of us just don't want to take the extra time during a busy day to explain why that prescription for a narcotic isn't a good idea. Some of us also use the promise of prescription narcotics to persuade patients to keep their medical appointments or to take their other medications.

It's important to take patients' pain seriously. Musculoskeletal disorders like back pain are among the top causes of disability in the U.S., but there are other ways to treat pain. Physical and chiropractic therapy, massage, and acupuncture aren't used enough, in part because they may be more expensive. Patients also don't want to have to wait for a referral or repeated treatments to get pain relief. Perhaps the best way to address pain is a team approach, in which primary-care doctors, pain specialists, physical therapists, chiropractors, acupuncturists; massage therapists, mental-health providers, and addiction specialist's work together to find the best solution for a shared patient.

Under the F.D.A. proposal, slated to take effect as early as next year, doctors would no longer be allowed to write six-month prescriptions for products like Vicodin that combine hydrocodone with over-the-counter painkillers. Instead, doctors could prescribe only a ninety-day supply of hydrocodone without a return visit. Earlier this year, the F.D.A. also recommended that prescription narcotics be made more abuse-resistant; it is blocking the approval of generic OxyContin that doesn't use this technology. And it requires that extended-release and long-acting forms of prescription narcotics be labeled to indicate that these medications are for "around-the-clock" severe pain and that alternative treatments should be considered first.

Those actions come as states and other local jurisdictions also crack down on the overprescribing of narcotics. Florida, for instance, passed a law making it illegal for anyone other than a doctor in good standing to run a pain clinic and limiting how much narcotic medication can be dispensed at one time. And many states are also now requiring physicians to police their patients by looking them up in online registries to ensure that they aren't "doctor-shopping" to get narcotics from multiple sources.

How Can Chiropractic Make A Difference With The Pain Pill Epidemic?

Pain pill addiction is becoming an epidemic among all segments of society but especially among teenagers. While illicit drug use (like marijuana, coke, etc.) is going down, prescription drug use is on the rise. This type of drug is extremely addictive when it is taken without proper medical supervision. Sometimes the problem begins after someone is given a pain pill prescription by their doctor after an injury or surgery and then they start to take them outside of the doctor's recommended dosing instructions.

Beyond the risks of addiction and overdose, prescription drugs that numb pain may convince a patient that a musculoskeletal condition is less severe than it is or that it has healed. This misunderstanding can lead to overexertion and a delay in the healing process or even permanent injury. Chiropractic and other conservatives (non-drug) approaches to pain management can be an important first line of defense against pain and addiction caused by the overuse of prescription opioid pain medications.

Rising Recognition of the Value of Non-drug Approaches to Pain

There is a growing body of research that validates the effectiveness of chiropractic services, leading many respected healthcare organizations to recommend chiropractic and its drug-free approach to pain relief.

In 2017, the American College of Physicians (ACP) updated its guidelines for the treatment of acute and chronic low back pain to recommend first using non-invasive, non-drug treatments before resorting to drug therapies. ACP's guidelines cite heat therapy, massage, acupuncture and spinal manipulation (a centerpiece of chiropractic care) as possible options for non-invasive, non-drug therapies for low back pain. Only when such treatments provide little or no relief, the guidelines state, should patients move on to medicines such as ibuprofen or muscle relaxants, which research indicates have limited pain-relief effects.

In March 2016, the Centers for Disease Control and Prevention, in response to the opioid epidemic, released guidelines for prescribing opioids that also promote non-pharmacologic alternatives for the treatment of chronic pain. In 2015, the Joint Commission, the organization that accredits more than 20,000 health care systems in the U.S. (including every major hospital), recognized the value of non-drug approaches by adding chiropractic and acupuncture to its pain management standard.

The American Chiropractic Association (ACA) encourages patients and health care providers to first exhaust conservative forms of pain management, when appropriate, before moving on to riskier, potentially addictive treatments such as opioids. To this end, ACA delegates met in Washington, D.C., in 2016 and adopted a policy statement proposing a solution to the dual public health concerns of inadequate pain management and opioid abuse.

How to Treat Prescription Opioid Addiction

Although prescription drug use and addiction are prevalent throughout the United States, so are resources to help. New legislation and guidelines are being implemented to reduce the proliferation of prescription opioids for minor issues. While they can be helpful and even life-saving for those suffering from severe pain, some types of chronic pain can be managed without opioids. Consult your doctor to learn more about other methods of pain management. Some alternatives to prescription opioids for chronic pain include:

- Acupuncture
- Physical therapy
- Massage therapy
- Daily yoga or other exercise practices
- Injections

For those who are addicted to prescription painkillers, however, overcoming physical and mental dependence can be a struggle. There are several options for those suffering from prescription drug addiction. Some options for overcoming opioid addiction include:

- Medical detox
- Comprehensive inpatient care programs
- Local outpatient therapy
- Medically assisted treatment
- Individual or family counseling
- Cognitive behavioral therapy

If you are ready to take the first step toward healing from prescription opioid addiction. With the help of dedicated and compassionate medical professionals, you can find the tools you need to overcome substance use disorder and enjoy a life free from the adverse effects of prescription opioid use.

Conclusion

Everyone has a role to play in curbing the spread of prescription drug abuse. Creating awareness about not using opioids beyond the prescribed limit, not sharing prescriptions with others and disposing of unused medicines, etc. will help to a great extent. As parents and guardians, there should be a constant tab on children about their unusual activities. Opioids prescriptions should be kept away from their reach.

CHAPTER 2: APPRECIATING THE MIRACLE OF LIFE

Before I discuss anything else, I want to take this chapter to begin to appreciate this thing called human life, appreciate the astounding way in which our human body works. I am not talking about something mystical. Instead, I'm asking you to think about the complexities of our body and isn't it marvelous that we exist in the first place. OUR BODIES ARE AMAZING!

Just think about our body that is made of billions and billions of cells working in sync with each other, the heart that beats untiringly 100, 000 times a day, our breath and senses which send millions of signals each day. Blood vessels extend thousands of miles and yet at the end of the day not a single breakdown. The key to changing our life is by first appreciating it.

Our life is marvelous! Everything is marvelous about the way we take shape from day one. Our brain is the first organ that starts forming; Then it is covered by the bony shield we call a skull in adults, after which our spinal cord, the powerful information highway starts developing. Only once the central computing and information highway is ready, do the other body parts, along with the organs start taking shape. The autonomic nervous system takes over the control of our internal organs, ensuring that heart beats as intended and digestive juices are secreted as required.

I am not trying to teach you human anatomy, but just to underline the intricacies of the human body. I am emphasizing the importance of the nervous system, and how it controls the functioning of each and every cell, playing a crucial role in health maintenance by responding to every challenge.

However, if our nervous system somehow fails to respond to these daily challenges suitably, the balance is broken. Yes, you've got it; it leads to disease. So, you must be asking in what way can I take control this process?

Summarizing the answer in one sentence: **Doctor's don't cure, the body cures itself.**

The good doctor is one who adopts a holistic approach and appreciates the flow of the healing power inside each of us.

So, what I want you to do right now is to thank your body in serving you in such a beautiful manner, appreciate your body for your existence and respect your body for doing all the wonderful things needed for your existence. Respect and appreciate the abilities of your body and treat it as most wonderful thing you have ever owned.

Realize what a wonderful gift your body is; there is a reason for you being here. You cannot get a kind of life you want without a true connection to the importance of your wellbeing. Start today with a new gratitude that your life requires true energy, not just a halfhearted effort. Aim for the maximum you have ever desired.

INNATE INTELLIGENCE AND THE BODY'S FUNCTIONS

As I already mentioned earlier, that the body starts with a single cell. But how is that single cell transformed into the massive body? Miracle?

Well, not exactly. This process is what Chiropractors have been calling *Innate Intelligence* for more than a century. Innate Intelligence is something that is created at the moment of your conception; it flows through your body. It is what makes your body function in a way it should be functioning without a glitch. Our body is a wonder of Innate Intelligence. It operates automatically. It does everything from maintaining your heart rhythm to keeping your skin supple.

THE LUNGS

Lungs are another brilliant example of Innate Intelligence at work. The primary function of lungs is to keep your body oxygenated, remove carbon dioxide and other wastes of metabolism. During inhalation, our rib cage expands to allow maximum air inside, while during exhalation rib cage becomes smaller to push out the air. Ribs are quite dynamic and muscles between them are flexible, allowing air to flow in and out of the lungs.

Though automatic, respiration is a highly regulated process, enabling our heart to breath 20-30,000 times a day and working continually under the supervision of the autonomous nervous system.

THE SKIN

Skin is not there just to provide the cover. In fact, it is the largest organ of our body amounting to about 16 percent of total body weight. Apart from protection, it helps to maintain body temperature, removes excess water, salt and toxins.

Skin is the first line of defense for our internal organs from every imaginable danger, be it infection or ultraviolet rays. Skin even converts sun rays to vitamin D and help to maintain healthy bones.

Skin also plays a vital role in communication, sensation, expression of emotions and even sexual attraction. It is made up of two layers called epidermis and dermis. Skin can also absorb oily substances.

THE DIGESTIVE SYSTEM

Digestion starts in the mouth. From there, food reaches the stomach while passing through the pipe called the esophagus. Movement of food in the digestive system happens due to a rhythmic movement called peristalsis. It is an action that is similar to squeezing from one end to the other. Peristalsis is a brilliant example of Innate Intelligence at work.

THE EYES

Despite their small size, eyes are the most important sensory organ, with millions of cells that provide the sense of sight. Although eyes can perceive only red, yellow, blue, and black, they can differentiate between 300 trillion colors!

Sitting in the bony socket of the skull, each eye has a lens to focus light on the sensor called the retina. The retina sends visual information to the brain with the help of optical nerves. The small colored portion in the center of the eyes called the iris, controls the amount of light that can enter inside the eye. In bright light the pupil contracts, while in low light conditions they dilate to allow more light into the eyes.

Eyes are protected by eyelids and eyelashes. They blink on a regular interval to keep the upper layer of eyes moist.

All these activities in the eyes happen automatically due to innate intelligence.

THE HAND

We are the only species with opposing fingers and thumbs. Each hand is an amazing instrument powered by 13 muscles and has 27 bones for extra flexibility. Hands can carry out very delicate jobs like playing the keyboard and tough jobs like participating in rigorous sports.

A chiropractor is especially good at understanding and treating the pain related to carpal tunnel syndrome. As an example, one of my clients who already had an operation for this condition came to me, because the pain was not relieved by surgery. I could see that the pain of the client was due to a problem in the neck!

THE MUSCLES

There are whopping 650 muscles in our body, making all of our movements possible. They are made to do most complicated tasks like picking small objects with tweezers to more robust tasks like running a marathon. Muscles also help to protect the internal organs.

We may know a lot about the functioning of our muscles. To perform any tasks, muscles must work in synchronization with various other organs. Moving from one place to another involves communication between muscles, ears, eyes and brain. <u>This internal communication happens by using the information highway called our nervous system.</u>

When our muscles and joints are moving, all the information about actions, movement, location is being transmitted to the brain at a subconscious level, but this communication is controlled by innate intelligence.

In fact, we do far more tasks than we ever realize. Thus, if a person starts talking to you, you automatically turn your head, eyes and start listening.

It is Innate Intelligence that makes **balancing** possible, by controlling the minor muscular movements at all times. Our balance and movement will become sluggish if even one small muscle fails to perform as required. Thus, the brain has to keep correcting the movement at all times.

THE SKELETAL SYSTEM

Without bones we would be just an enormous blob with no shape or structure. We would not be able to stand or walk. Without bones, we would be just a pile of skin, muscles, and guts.

Our skeletal system is made up of <u>206 bones</u>, designed to be strong, and to protect our body. <u>At birth we have 300 bones</u>, but as we grow many of them fuse together.

Bones have many functions. <u>The spinal vertebrae not only protect the information highway</u> but also help us to stand erect and walk upright. Bones protect the delicate internal organs. Just consider the skull. It's like a strong helmet safeguarding our brain. The rib cage protects our heart and lungs.

Unlike the common perception that bones are cold and inert, they are in fact, very dynamic. Bones are made of a hard layer for providing strength and cells that help them grow and repair. That is why if you have ever broken your arm or leg, it heals.

Apart from mechanical support and protection, bones are also responsible for producing red and white blood cells. Red blood cells are responsible for carrying oxygen to body tissues, while white blood cells are the part of the immune system, thus helping to protect our body from infections and diseases.

ONCE AGAIN... THE NERVOUS SYSTEM IS AMAZING!

We once again return to discuss the system that controls our majestic body- the nervous system. It consists of the brain, spinal cord and peripheral nerves. <u>The brain is the main computing center</u> that sends signals to various parts of the body, performing billions of operations, yet consuming merely around ten watts of energy. <u>The spinal cord is the information "Superhighway," that is responsible for distributing all the information.</u> Spinal nerves are the exit points of the highway.

<u>The nervous system is operated by the Innate Intelligence</u> that is vital for the functioning of every cell. And most of the time, it efficiently performs its tasks to ensure that the body works in tandem. Innate intelligence can be called the "internal divine guidance" that overlooks all the critical function to ensure proper health.

Any disruption in communication between the body parts and the brain would lead to either pain or a loss of functionality. It is like a disruption in the telephone line which compromises communication between two parties.

Conclusion

For optimal health, it is vital that our nervous system is working correctly all the time to maintain hundred percent communication throughout the body. In this chapter, we demonstrated that our body is made up of various systems that operate in synchronization with each other to ensure optimal health. Under the guidance of Innate Intelligence.

CHAPTER 3: WHAT IS "HEALTH?"

Suppose that I were to ask you to define the term "health." What kind of answer would you give me? There is a general opinion and consensus that good health is: (1) feeling "fine," or (2) when everything is working okay, or (3) when there is an absence of pain.

All of these definitions are partial and are far from complete. Taber's medical dictionary defines health as, "A condition in which all functions of the body and mind are normally active." The World Health Organization defines health as a state of complete physical, mental or social well-being and not merely the absence of disease or infirmity. So the next question to ask is how does one quantify health? In a sense then, health is equal to balance. How do you determine balance? What are the determining factors in the balancing equation? To answer this we must first ask, what comprises the overall scheme of health? Also, what kind of an overall gauge can be used to reflect back on the quality of health we experience or lack there of?

In order to get to the core of good health you need to start at the cellular level. The balancing act begins there. You see the quality of your life is based on the quality of the life of your cells. Considering the fact that you are comprised of over 70 trillion cells, you can assume that when those cells are working optimally in perfect harmony with each other, you will have health. But again how does one quantify this?

Now if health equals balance, then we can state that the opposite of health, which is not disease, but rather dis-ease meaning a lack of balance or ease. It can also be said that the cells are not functioning correctly.

Raymond Francis, a chemist and graduate of MIT, believes through his research that there is only one reason in which disease is created. That reason is simply due to cells not functioning properly. When you think about that statement, it makes sense. Now there are only two reasons why cells do not function appropriately. They are:

1. Cells are not receiving proper nutrition and/or
2. Cells are not eliminating their toxicity produced by the normal functioning of the cell.

Now there are at the root many reasons why these cells can become dysfunctional. Those reasons are:

- Lack of appropriate levels of oxygen
- Lack of nutrients
- The inability to eliminate waste
- Improper nerve impulse to the cell

To begin to understand this process let us quickly visit the stages of health. When one is conceived, we are given as a birthright the ability to express health effortlessly. However if there is a disturbance in the intimate relationship between the nervous system and the rest of the body, you will lose your efficient ability to express health.

As we age, we experience the effects of the years initially only through a microscopic inspection. Long before we feel the effects of age, our cells are beginning to experience changes. Cells are beginning to replicate less efficiently, and then one day we transition from the anabolic phase of life, which means that sufficient cells are replacing those that have just died, to a phase of catabolic metabolism, in which we have more cells that are dying than are being replaced. When we enter the catabolic stage, we must do everything within our power to slow it down.

To better understand the process of health, it helps to understand the phases of health. The first phase is one of perfect balance or homeostasis. This is optimal health where everything is working the way it was designed to work. However, as we age, we begin to encounter emotional, physical, and chemical stresses in our lives to the point where we will enter into a phase of imbalance, lack of ease, or dis-ease. Health can easily be regained in this phase as long as we refocus our efforts on finding the cause of what brought us initially on that path of imbalance. If that is achieved, then we can regain a state of balance.

However, if this phase is not dealt with appropriately, then we enter into a phase of discomfort, and dis-ease. This phase can have with it associated levels of pain, but not in all cases. Sometime there are no visible or felt symptoms. If we stay in this phase for any real amount of time, we begin to have dis-ease of more than one cell. It begins to affect thousands and thousands of cells, to the point of reaching into the body's tissues. Left further without a reversal of the dis-ease, then it enters into a larger group of tissues which would then be affecting organs. It then moves onto systems, and then ultimately it affects the entire being, and we then die.

I'm not proposing that we can live forever. I am however saying that 90% of our medical expense is spent during the last 10% of our lives. People are no longer dying of natural causes. The majority of deaths in this country are related to degenerative processes. When one can minimize that process one can live a longer, higher quality of life.

Therefore, the key to overall health is to correctly determine the appropriate factors involved in health. This means managing health at the cellular level. Health is a consequence of choices one has made or not made.

A Doctor's Approach to Health

Imagine going to a doctor when you had nothing wrong with you. Your blood pressure was fine, your cholesterol was reasonable, your weight was appropriate for your age and height. What if at this visit you told the doctor that all you wanted to do was maintain this? Hopefully he or she would say, "great," but they may not be able to offer you much more in the way of maintenance than to say, "keep on doing whatever you are doing." The point here is that that kind of advice would only work for so long. That is because the medical system is at best designed for the early detection of disease, but not for the prevention.

How would you react to a mechanic that told you that all you need to do for your car is bring it in and have the oil changed when the car starts to give you problems? We all know what that would do, don't we? We know what the consequences of not getting an oil change on time does to our car, which incidentally we will only have for 10 years at best, and yet we don't always give our bodies that we will hopefully have for many decades, the same kind of preventative care.

Antibiotics & Dis-Ease

Why do we put so little effort into maintaining our bodies? That is because most people believe that there is a magic pill that will solve all of our problems. Again no medicine has ever cured anyone. The body does the healing; it happens no other way.

The birth of medicine could be attributed to the time when Robert Koch postulated the germ theory in 1860. Once this discovery took place, it was therefore emphasized and widely believed that microbes were the cause of disease. It was also widely accepted that the key to health was to destroy those foreign enemies.

This theory has resulted in the overuse of antibiotics to the point that we are now dealing with super-strains of bacteria and viruses. These microbes are becoming more and more resistant to all of the antibiotics originally created to fight them off.

Alternative Health Options

People today are becoming more and more aware of alternatives. They are sick and tired of being sick and tired and they want options. They want to know why they are sick or why they are feeling a certain way. They are sick and tired of hearing obscure explanations on what they have and why taking a "magic pill" will solve all their problems.

We are getting smarter. In the United States in the year 2001 there were more visits to Alternative Health Care practitioners than traditional allopathic medical doctors. It may have started with the baby boomers who wanted to create and maintain health, not just mask their problems with drugs and surgery. We are not being attacked by the flu. We are not innocent victims being chosen by microbes. We are in fact creating the very environment for these bacteria and viruses to feast upon a body that is full of toxicity -- the perfect environment in which bacteria and viruses thrive.

Anyone can change their attitude and approach to health. If you continue to look at your body the same way you have in the past, you will continue to get what you have gotten in the past. However, if you want to change things, start with your mindset. You must prioritize your health as not something that should be tolerated, but something that must be maintained and even improved. In life, it seems we only do consistently that which we find important enough to make a priority. It is important, therefore, to look at your health as something that is so important that it becomes top priority.

To make your health a priority you must realize that there are a variety of different choices we make everyday that can be categorized into two broad areas: Doing things that are important and urgent; and doing things that are important and not urgent.

Everything in your life that adds meaning to your life and fulfillment to it, such as spending time with your family, spending time giving thanks to your creator, working out, eating the right foods, spending quality time with your significant other, are all under the category of things that are important but not urgent. In order for you to create the highest level of health possible, you must consistently focus on doing things in the area of health that are important for you.

The question to ask your self is, "What can I do today to start on a path of wellness?" I recommend that my patients make the changes that are very easy to do. For example, I had a patient who had not exercised in many, many years. I asked her if she could spend 5 minutes a day just stretching. Of course that sounded very easy to do. Before long, that 5 minute stretch turned into 10 minutes. Next, she realized that the stretching really felt good and added some light resistance to her routine with some hand weights. By the end of a month, she had added the cardiovascular to the routine and was up to a half hour of exercising. It felt so good that the habit was one she intended on maintaining.

You see once you create a habit, you can expand upon it, but you will set yourself up for failure if you start too big. The most important thing that I want you to get out of this chapter is the subtle consequences our choices have on our health. There are small decisions we make everyday that can make the difference between being completely well or not.

If you would like to test out this theory for yourself, I have an assignment for you. First, get yourself a health journal. It can be any small notebook that you can keep with you. Next, write down the following on the inside cover or first page of your journal:

"I hereby grant myself permission to bring my health to the highest level I was meant to experience, by nurturing myself, by taking care of myself, and by forgiving myself as I would a loved one. I declare today, a day that I will never forget, for it is the day that my life and health was changed forever."

Your health journal should begin with a list of goals. These can categorized as physical, mental and spiritual. You may want to eat better, so be specific and list the types of foods you will avoid to obtain better health. If you want to learn a new skill or improve a relationship, list specific actions you can take and over which you have complete control. The more specific you are the more successful you will be.

Each day, record in your journal or notebook the small steps you have taken. Record even your set backs and shortcomings because those will help you see the progress you are making over time.

How can chiropractic care effect your health?

The biggest way Chiropractic can help you is by number one not focusing on symptoms, but rather on the body's ability to regain health. If you always chase symptoms, you will never truly regain your body's health potential. You will always be days or months away from your next symptom, and you will be focused on relieving those symptoms as quickly as possible.

Being under chiropractic care allows you to change your perception of going to the doctor only when there is a problem to going to the chiropractor because you don't want to have any problems in the future.

Where would we be if we had a health care system in which the doctors were only paid based on how healthy their patients are? Sound crazy? That's exactly what is happening in Japan. Doctor's get paid based on how healthy their patients are. It does not impress me whatsoever, when a doctor says that it's a good thing that you came in because we just found some major problems in you, and we need to go in immediately for a bypass, or something equally invasive. Problems like that just don't appear out of nowhere. It takes years and years for conditions to develop and get to that point. Again we have technology within the medical community that emphasizes early detection at best and very little, if any, prevention.

You can't just blame the doctors here either. It is the responsibility of each individual to care for themselves and to take action to prevent disease. It is the responsibility of every parent to see that their children are on a path of good, life long health through preventative care.

How can Chiropractic be a strategy to attain health?

The science of chiropractic is in and of itself a fundamental strategy for good health. When you are under chiropractic care, you work to reduce any stress or strain around the spine which in turn could affect the body's ability to adapt to all that is thrown its way.

You see, if there is any kind of interference within or surrounding the nervous system it causes dis-ease or creates a situation where you are not completely well. Often that interference can't be felt. There may no pain or pressure at all to tell you something isn't right. Rather the only thing you experience from this is the effects of it. Sadly, it may take months or even years for the symptoms to manifest themselves.

This might be easier to understand if you use the example of breast cancer. Did you know that it takes years to create enough density within the breast tissue in order to see a tumor growth via X-ray? By that time it may be too late.

Chiropractic does not emphasize waiting for something to go wrong, and then coming in as the hero to only remove the symptom, doing very little about the actual cause of the problem. It focuses on maintaining your natural state of wellness at an optimal level of existence, so that you are at the highest level neurologically speaking.

Think about it this way: if you applied the same rationale to your life in every aspect, would it make your life better or richer, or would it make it worse? If you applied the preventative model to your finances, what would it do? If you applied it to your relationship with your spouse, what would that do? All the areas of your life would see a marked improvement. You would no longer be waiting for things to get to the point of being urgent. You would be proactive instead of reactive. You are prioritizing your health as being important while not waiting for a crisis to make changes.

How Chiropractic Can Change Your Life

The system I propose is based on a true mind body approach that I call the IE technology – or Information and Empowerment. You see with information and empowerment, you can truly make a difference in your life. Here is a summary of the key factors needed to sustain health. More details are provided in the chapters on nutrition and exercise.

The first aspect of the system involves beliefs. You must first create the mental construct that will allow you to filter a reality with which you want to be congruent. In other words, you must believe in things that you want to have happen.

Next, is to understand the importance of exercise. You must exercise. It is not an option, and you can't justify not exercising because you already work hard at work, you already chase the kids around the house, and you already work in the garden. All of these activities are a good start to movement, but do not constitute a real workout. You must have a cardiovascular workout for health – one that challenges and works your heart. Remember your heart is a muscle and it needs to pump a lot of blood through your entire body every day for a very long time. You must challenge it so it can be as strong as possible.

The third aspect of this equation is the importance of breathing correctly. You must provide oxygen to the tissues of the body. If you don't, you will have problems because they will suffocate. Oxygen supplies and nourishes not only the lungs, but every cell within the body. The lungs are just the clearinghouse.

The fourth important factor is drinking water. This is necessary in order to flush out toxins from the body. After all your body is 75% water; not 75% coffee, or tea, or soda. These drinks just give you an illusion of energy. There is no sustaining power behind any of them, even though the caffeine addict may object to this statement.

The next fundamental truth relates to greens. Most people do not understand the magnitude of the importance of greens. Eating enough green, leafy vegetables each week is one of the most powerful things you can do for yourself. Think about this, to understand why plants are so necessary to good health. When plants are outside, they convert light into energy, in the process known as photosynthesis. Through this amazing process, we are able to literally consume energy through the plants.

Most importantly, you must consume some raw vegetables, or you are totally defeating the purpose. Raw plants contain the necessary enzymes that are often destroyed by over cooking. Enzymes are vital to good health.

The next nutrient that you need to have is antioxidants. Antioxidants allow you to minimize the ravaging effects of free radicals that are within us and increase in number as we age. Free radicals are produced in times of stress, during injury, or during chemical processes that are taking place due to the consumption of processed foods. Free radicals left to roam can cause damage right at the cellular level. Damaged cells lead to a lowered immune system and increase the likelihood of infection and disease.

The next dietary items you need to have are fats and oils. Fats are needed to assure that your body has sufficient levels of oil to make the cell membrane of the cell. This outer layer of the cell is made of a double layer called a biphospholipid layer.

The problem with fats and oils in the diet is that many of us consume too much or the wrong type of fats. According to researchers, the average person is deficient in correct oil consumption by up to 90%! That is staggering considering the connection between low levels of essential oils in our diets and cardiovascular disease and the resulting list of degenerative disorders. So, believe it or not, oils are by far the best preventative measure that you can take.

The last pro-active step you that you need to take is to maintain a healthy nervous system. Think about this for a moment. If you were consuming everything that I recommended, and yet your nervous system was not functioning properly, how would the brain tell the cells what to do with the nutrients it just received? How would the brain contact the cell to let it know when to remove waste?

Consider this research from a professor by the name of Professor Tzu. He claims that pressure put on a nerve with the weight of only a dime can interfere with normal transmission of impulse by up to 60%! It is staggering how little pressure it takes to reduce you body's own ability to send corrective, healing messages by so much.

CHAPTER 4: THE HEALTH MODEL VS. THE SICK MODEL

One important and positive way that health care is changing is that it's moving from a "sick care" model to a "well care" model. What does this mean? Well, in years past, most health care was provided on a reactive basis. Meaning when you got sick, you went to the doctor; this is the "sick care" model. Today healthcare is moving toward a "well care" model, in which a proactive approach is taken instead, through an ongoing relationship with a primary care practitioner (PCP).

The Health Model (also known as the wellness model) is a theory in caring for clients and patients that take the focus from being sick to preventative care. In the wellness model, there is a strong emphasis on holistic care where the client or patient is encouraged to take part in healthy activities that create a stronger body and mind that can ward off illness, instead of relying on the traditional health system to care for a sick body. Wellness is not just a set of practices that are incorporated at the doctor's office, but rather it's a change in lifestyle. Wellness includes care from your regular physician but also can include chiropractic, massage, nutrition, fitness and mental health care. All of these things make you a healthier person.

Health Care vs. Sick Care

Health care is wellness. It's everything that helps you move towards health and prevent problems from occurring again or even in the first place. This includes things like nutrition, exercise, whole food supplements, dental care, chiropractic care, massage, and acupuncture.

Think of it this way. Imagine a spectrum. Health is on one end of the spectrum, and sickness is on the other end of the spectrum. Your position on this spectrum can shift toward one side or the other depending on several factors. On the health end of the spectrum, the focus is on prevention and being proactive in doing things to promote and support health. On the sick end, the focus is on addressing the crisis and being reactive to the disease or illness.

Sick care is damage control. The obvious need for "sick care" is in emergency situations, such as accidents, traumas, and other life-or-death acute conditions. Management of chronic conditions like heart disease, cancer, and diabetes is also included in "sick care." The main goal of "sick care" is to stop you from getting worse. The secondary goal is to make you feel better but not necessarily correct the cause of your problem. The "sick care" model rarely focuses on moving you back towards health and preventing the problem from occurring again.

The Wellness Approach

Wellness care seeks to turn on the natural healing ability, not by adding something to the system, but by removing anything that might interfere with normal function, trusting that the body would know what to do if nothing were interfering with it. Standard medical care, on the other hand, seeks to treat a symptom by adding something from the outside - a medication, a surgery or procedure.

Wellness is a state of optimal conditions for normal function... and then some. The wellness approach is to look for underlying causes of any disturbance or disruption (which may or may not be causing symptoms at the time) and make whatever interventions and lifestyle adjustments would optimize the conditions for normal function. That environment encourages natural healing, and minimizes the need for invasive treatment, which should be administered only when absolutely necessary. When the body is working properly, it tends to heal effectively, no matter what the condition. When the body heals well and maintains itself well, then there is another level of health that goes beyond "asymptomatic" or "pain-free" which reveals an open-ended opportunity for vitality, vibrant health, and an enhanced experience of life. This is true for mental and emotional health as well as physical health. While some people may suffer psychological disorders, creating an atmosphere of mental and emotional wellness will address all but the most serious problems.

The Concepts Of Illness Behavior And Sick-Role Behavior In Healthcare

Generally, health-related behaviors of healthy people and those who try to maintain their health are considered as behaviors related to primary prevention of disease. Such behaviors are intended to reduce susceptibility to disease, as well as to reduce the effects of chronic diseases when they occur in the individual. Secondary prevention of disease is more closely related to the control of a disease that an individual has or that is incipient in the individual. This type of prevention is most closely tied to illness behavior. Tertiary prevention is generally seen as directed towards reducing the impact and progression of symptomatic disease in the individual. This type of prevention is highly related to the concept of sick-role behavior.

In present-day public health practice, which is based on population and community-based approaches with an emphasis on participation, the research from these concepts of behavior has helped immensely in clarifying critical approaches to public health. The concept of diversity in populations has been greatly enhanced through the articulation of the concepts of illness behavior and the sick role.

Researchers now have a significant body of research showing the wide variation in these behaviors with respect to all the key demographic variables. For example, there has been excellent work showing how the presentation of symptoms to a physician is highly dependent on gender, ethnic background, and other socio-cultural characteristics. Research on the sick-role concept has elucidated the issue of power and its many manifestations in doctors' offices, hospitals, and other medical settings. It would be difficult, given this literature, for a practicing health educator not to consider the role of power in patient-physician interactions.

In general, illness and sick-role behaviors are viewed as characteristics of individuals and as concepts derived from sociological and socio-psychological theories.

Illness Behavior

The concept of illness behavior was largely defined and adopted during the second half of the twentieth century. Broadly speaking, it is any behavior undertaken by an individual who feels ill to relieve that experience or to better define the meaning of the illness experience. There are many different types of illness behavior that have been studied. Some individuals who experience physical or mental symptoms turn to the medical care system for help; others may turn to self-help strategies; while others may decide to dismiss the symptoms.

In everyday life, illness behavior may be a mixture of behavioral decisions. For example, an individual faced with recurring symptoms of joint pain may turn to complementary or alternative medicine for relief. However, sudden, sharp, debilitating symptoms may lead one directly to a hospital emergency room. In any event, illness behavior is usually mediated by strong subjective interpretations of the meaning of symptoms. As with any type of human behavior, many social and psychological factors intervene and determine the type of illness behavior expressed in the individual.

The Health Belief Model

The Health Belief Model (HBM) was developed in the early 1950s by social scientists at the U.S. Public Health Service in order to understand the failure of people to adopt disease prevention strategies or screening tests for the early detection of disease. Later uses of HBM were for patients' responses to symptoms and compliance with medical treatments. The HBM suggests that a person's belief in a personal threat of an illness or disease together with a person's belief in the effectiveness of the recommended health behavior or action will predict the likelihood the person will adopt the behavior.

The Health Belief Model is a framework for motivating people to take positive health actions that uses the desire to avoid a negative health consequence as the prime motivation. For example, HIV is a negative health consequence, and the desire to avoid HIV can be used to motivate sexually active people into practicing safe sex. Similarly, the perceived threat of a heart attack can be used to motivate a person with high blood pressure into exercising more often.

It's important to note that avoiding a negative health consequence is a key element of the HBM. For example, a person might increase exercise to look good and feel better. That example does not fit the model because the person is not motivated by a negative health outcome — even though the health action of getting more exercise is the same as for the person who wants to avoid a heart attack.

The HBM derives from psychological and behavioral theory with the foundation that the two components of health-related behavior are the desire to avoid illness, or conversely get well if already ill; and the belief that a specific health action will prevent, or cure, illness. Ultimately, an individual's course of action often depends on the person's perceptions of the benefits and barriers related to health behavior. There are six constructs of the HBM.

Perceived Susceptibility: This refers to a person's subjective perception of the risk of acquiring an illness or disease. There is wide variation in a person's feelings of personal vulnerability to an illness or disease.

Perceived Severity: This refers to a person's feelings on the seriousness of contracting an illness or disease (or leaving the illness or disease untreated). There is wide variation in a person's feelings of severity, and often a person considers the medical consequences (e.g., death, disability) and social consequences (e.g., family life, social relationships) when evaluating the severity.

Perceived Benefits: This refers to a person's perception of the effectiveness of various actions available to reduce the threat of illness or disease (or to cure illness or disease). The course of action a person takes in preventing (or curing) illness or disease relies on consideration and evaluation of both perceived susceptibility and perceived benefit, such that the person would accept the recommended health action if it was perceived as beneficial.

Perceived Barriers: This refers to a person's feelings on the obstacles to performing a recommended health action. There is wide variation in a person's feelings of barriers, or impediments, which lead to a cost/benefit analysis. The person weighs the effectiveness of the actions against the perceptions that it may be expensive, dangerous (e.g., side effects), unpleasant (e.g., painful), time-consuming, or inconvenient.

Cue To Action: This is the stimulus needed to trigger the decision-making process to accept a recommended health action. These cues can be internal (e.g., chest pains, wheezing, etc.) or external (e.g., advice from others, illness of family member, newspaper article, etc.).

Self-Efficacy: This refers to the level of a person's confidence in his or her ability to successfully perform a behavior. This construct was added to the model most recently in mid-1980. Self-efficacy is a construct in many behavioral theories as it directly relates to whether a person performs the desired behavior.

Limitations of Health Belief Model

There are several limitations of the HBM which limit its utility in public health. Limitations of the model include the following:

- It does not account for a person's attitudes, beliefs, or other individual determinants that dictate a person's acceptance of a health behavior.
- It does not take into account behaviors that are habitual and thus may inform the decision-making process to accept a recommended action (e.g., smoking).
- It does not take into account behaviors that are performed for non-health related reasons such as social acceptability.

- It does not account for environmental or economic factors that may prohibit or promote the recommended action.
- It assumes that everyone has access to equal amounts of information on the illness or disease.
- It assumes that cues to action are widely prevalent in encouraging people to act and that "health" actions are the main goal in the decision-making process.

The HBM is more descriptive than explanatory, and does not suggest a strategy for changing health-related actions. In preventive health behaviors, early studies showed that perceived susceptibility, benefits, and barriers were consistently associated with the desired health behavior; perceived severity was less often associated with the desired health behavior. The individual constructs are useful, depending on the health outcome of interest, but for the most effective use of the model, it should be integrated with other models that account for the environmental context and suggest strategies for change.

Preventative Healthcare

Health is a state of wholeness in which your body knows its ever-changing needs and responds to those, all on its own. Inside Out Chiropractic believes that chiropractic care is a long-term form of preventative healthcare that maintains your body's nervous system to keep you in good health for a lifetime.

True chiropractic care in a principled practice believes that bodily health exists when the body is in a state of wholeness; it understands its own constantly-changing needs, and is able to respond to them on its own. Chiropractic care doesn't heal injuries; rather, it helps the body to engage its own incredible natural healing abilities through a long-term routine of preventative healthcare maintenance for the nervous system.

Preventative healthcare focuses on your entire nervous system: your brain, spinal cord, and every one of the millions of nerve connections throughout your body. It monitors your entire body and all its needs, to help control and coordinate the necessary responses that allow the body to learn, adapt and constantly maintain its own health and wellness.

Preventative Care Vs. Sick Care

The common healthcare model in the United States is the sick care model. It only looks at your body after symptoms of illness present, and then considers how best to treat these symptoms.

The preventative healthcare chiropractic model, on the other hand, is entirely natural, non-invasive, doesn't rely on chemicals, and looks to the root cause of your underlying health issues. It is focused entirely on correcting spinal subluxations to allow your whole nervous system to communicate better and increase the body's overall healing abilities. This improves your ability to adapt to stress and a variety of health conditions and helps to restore you to normal, healthy and optimal function. Chiropractic can restore your natural healing capability, and provide increased vitality, energy, bodily functions and overall health.

Hospitals and the Wellness Sham

Furthermore, while hospitals and health systems may preach wellness, few offer comprehensive services designed to improve your health and well-being. Rather, they pay lip-service to this essential component of health care – viewing wellness more as a marketing opportunity than a true effort to do everything in their power to minimize unnecessary and costly utilization of their medical services.

There's no surprise here, since the dominant reimbursement mechanism, the fee for service, rewards the provision of medical services – not maximization of the health of a defined population. As a result, we pay a very dear price.

How to Move from Sickness to Wellness

This can be a big challenge for some of our clients. And the reality is, moving from a sickness state of mind to a wellness state of mind is incredibly personal. It is possible to shift from a sick-care system that doles out interventions to manage the burden of chronic illness to a positive health system, focused on wellness/well-being system that minimizes unnecessary utilization by focusing on population health. However, it would require tremendous will on the part of numerous constituents to achieve such a powerful transformation.

The key to transitioning from one model to the other is time and support. When we meet a new client who can benefit from the wellness model, we address their immediate issues, and then create a positive and encouraging atmosphere that they can feel comfortable expanding into. If they've come to see us for chiropractic care, we may encourage them to support that function with a visit to one of our massage therapists or a fitness class. Treating the whole body with kindness and mindfulness is often all it takes to move a client from being "sick" to being "well."

Far short of transformational change, there are nonetheless small seeds of hope in the form of new, evolving reimbursement and delivery models, such as ACOs and medical homes that stress population health management. Unfortunately, the pace of adoption is glacial. For providers who have been burned in the past by assuming the risk for a defined population, there's little enthusiasm for doing so again.

Our Role in Changing the System

More than three decades ago, Jim Fries gave us one of the keys to healing American health care; a silver bullet. The question is whether we have the fortitude to change the healthcare paradigm, as well as accept the personal, stewardship responsibility for our health that is essential to success. Below are the roles for each of us to play:

Government: There needs to be dramatically increased spending on proven prevention programs that can be administered at a local, state, or federal level. Furthermore, there need to be greater rewards under governmental reimbursement programs for those providers who embrace risk and demonstrate their ability to reduce the morbidity of a defined population.

Consumers/Patients: We need to understand what it means to be prudent stewards of our health, and the health of our families. It is essential that we understand the role lifestyle choices make in determining our health, and how we might combat risk-factors that imperil our future. For many of us, we will need to have access to resources that will aid in this journey – particularly if we are socio-economically challenged, and thus find lifestyle change all the more difficult. As has been well-demonstrated, the social determinants of health play a profound role in wellness and well-being.

Providers: Healthcare executives need to take the moral high-ground and do the right things for the communities they serve. One place to begin is with the development of a strategic wellness plan illustrating how wellness initiatives can be integrated into the very fabric of your hospital or health system's care model. Once developed and implemented, you can then reasonably assert that you do everything possible to minimize unnecessary consumption of health care resources while maximizing the health and well-being of your patients.

Insurers/Payers: There needs to be an unremitting pressure to partner more fully with providers on the assumption of risk for the health and well-being of a defined population, thus accelerating the demise of fee-for-service medicine, and its replacement with a reimbursement mechanism that rewards wellness.

Employers: There needs to be broader adoption and implementation of wellness programs that incorporate proven mechanisms for elevating the health and well-being of an employed population. Such programs will likely involve potent incentives for lifestyle modification by those employees at risk.

Conclusion

It's time to put the "health" back in healthcare. Physicians must join with other health care practitioners whose focus is on building health and wellness and not just managing disease and illness. Drugs and surgeries target the main complaint and symptoms. But they fail to address the cause of the problems plaguing current day society. No amount of medication will address the true cause of degenerative diseases if the dysfunction within the body is not identified and restored. The irony is that the majority of the top 10 causes of death in modern society are rooted in diet and lifestyle (heart disease, certain cancers, diabetes, Alzheimer's – to name a few). These conditions may never have grown to their current epic proportions if the medical community would have continued to honor the fundamental health building values of diet and exercise.

CHAPTER 5: PHASES OF HEALING

In a former chapter, we have explained the chiropractic practices and how these can assist you and your system switch back to a healthy, optimal state. To comprehend better how this approach can aid in you in increasing your strength, health, and longevity, this section will be dedicated to the specific cycles of chiropractic healing. But before we jump onto this, we are going to affirm this statement--chiropractic practice isn't a fast cure or overnight miracle. If your system is out of whack, that is the result of years of issues to reach that unhealthy condition. While the good news is that, it won't take years to regain back your health, it will take some time for sure. Therefore, you need to practice patience and devotion. Let's now explain all the cycles, one after the other.

STAGE 1-THE INTENSE INFLAMMATORY PHASE

This is the stage that urges people to pay more attention and seek some type of expert help. This could be conventional medicine methods or alternative means, when everything else doesn't manage to bring the desired effects. Why is that? Simple because this pain is governed by its own pain and discomfort. Remember previously in this report where we dispelled the misconception that chiropractic practice was painful?? Chiropractic method in its nature is not painful. What actually triggers pain is your system's reaction to painful and sore tissue under work. Some of your joints and muscles are connected to be soft. Or perhaps your overall system is painful, which is a result of your own system's hypersensitivity to pain, as your body is subject to this pain for long periods of time.

This is the stage in which we chiropractors examine our patients because at this point, it is given that the patient experiences some level of pain or signs of discomfort like swelling, itchiness, redness, loss of balance and so on. The patients that come to visit us, are not doing so because they want to improve their health, but because they are fed-up of being in pain. Their main concern is to reduce their pain and symptoms and not the underlying mechanisms or origins of their issue.

It is vital to state here that this stage doesn't just happen overnight. It took ages and many years for your system to reach such a painful status and years of mishandling and doing inappropriate moves. So, as supported in this report, healing during this initial stage requires some time and can take up to 4 months to see good results. And anticipate that you'll have to come to a chiropractor's office once or twice a week. While this may sound a bit far to the ear's of the average american who wants a quick fix, it is actually a minimal investment for your long-term health.

It should be pointed out though, that therapy will vary in regards to power and frequency, based on the following factors:

- Sex
- Age
- Height
- Weight

- The time you've been suffering from this issue
- The level you are capable of following your physician's suggestions
- The max. pain level you can tolerate
- If and whether you experience other health problems

Upon the initial consultation, the chiropractor will assess all the above parameters as well as any other relevant aspects and problems, to come up with a personalized plan for your case. Your needs and challenges of course, will be also taken into account. However, this isn't like medicine--the chiropractic approach isn't the same for everyone.

STAGE 2-The RESTORATIVE AND CORRECTIVE STAGE

During this stage, you pain and discomfort issues will begin to subside. Your pain will become much more tolerable and while you won't feel as if you are running like a first-class athlete, you will most likely feel better and have a more positive mood. Sitting or standing will no longer be painful.

This is the point where we rely to rehabilitate strength and integrity and take off the damaged tissue that prevents the road to full and felt recovery. This a great stage as the patient starts to feel better. The energy levels of the patient start to increase and the scope of motion is restored. This is due to the fact that pain "eats" vast amounts of energy. So the logic of pain reduction to increase energy during this stage, has a point.

But there is one aspect that we need to pay extra attention to, during this cycle of treatment and this is to avoid pushing you and forcing you too early. Like most folks who get treated, you might mistakenly think that you can do everything you wish, after you've just begun to feel better. The issue is, if you push yourself too hard and do inappropriate movements, you may end up with worse pain than before, due to the fact that your initial issues that made you visit a chiropractor in the first place are still lingering in your system.

During this phase, our aim in chiropractic treatment is to concentrate our movements on the boost of spinal mobility so that the healthy physiological function is restored to your spine and nerves. You might still have to visit your physician once of week but this depends on the intensity of your condition.

Keep in mind that this correcting stage isn't a brief one, but there are other parameters and factors that can surely affect the speed of the healing progress. This can feature length of time and intensity of the issue. If, for instance, you come to the office after suffering from multiple car accidents in a row (yep, it might sound bizarre but I had a patient like this), of course, it will take much more time for the therapy to start working compared to the average patient that has poor posture problems intensified over the last few years. Some things that affect the therapy and slow down the progress are:

- Poor diet/nutrition
- Smoking
- Stress
- Improper ergonomics
- A negative mindset

We'll tackle some of these factors as we proceed with this section. (the only thing we won't address is smoking as there are countless of studies and evidence that proves the destructive effects of smoking and you don't need us to tell you so). In a later section, we will also to some basic nutrition guidelines to help speed up your recovery process. But at the moment, we are going to proceed to the next healing cycle.

STAGE III-THE MAINTENANCE STAGE

I love seeing this specific stage in a patient that visits me. This means that they have followed the treatment and there doing what they can do to restore their health and feel their best they have ever felt maybe in their life. The pain is minimized or at least kept under control.

Once the system achieves a state of health, it's necessary to maintain it. The good thing is that while you go through this phase, it's much easier to maintain your body to this healthy status. Remember that a status of perfect health, doesn't only imply lack of pain and disease-- it is a state of optimal physical, mental, and even interpersonal well-being. Once your system enjoys health, you will most probably feel the best you've felt for years.

Another advantage is that in this state of health, even if you are bothered by a spinal injury, it will recover more quickly and not many treatment sessions will be needed afterwards. Consider this: when a highly practiced and fit athlete endures an injury, he/she recovers more quickly than the average Joe (provided that the athlete doesn't push their limits to far and use the injured part more than they should). This is due to the fact they are used to conditioning practices and their systems are in optimal health already. Recovery, for this reason, is much faster.

Consider kids and the rate they recover from such injuries. This is due to the fact that our systems are wired from a very young age to recover and restore perfect health. As we grow older though and age, the rates of recovery start to slow down and we are less resistant and able to fight any health problems as quickly as young people. During the maintenance stage though, the system is loaded with more things to work with.

This stage goes more than a periodical chiropractic sessions, however. It boils down to lifetime habits and patterns. This where the majority of people begin to feel uncomfortable as this translates to more healthy diet, exercise, and a positive, stress-free mindset.

We hear many different excuses in our work (don't stress, we sometimes use these too as we are just humans). Perhaps the greatest excuse is lack of sufficient time. But, there is always some time to decide on what's vital in your life, what's your priority to achieve health. You should prioritize some things to make sure you take the matter of health in your own hands.

Nathaniel Branden, an inspiring psychologist who has authored many books about self-confidence and self-esteem, supports that the things we try to improve, are the things we already realize, while the areas that we neglect to work on, are the ones that we don't pay attention to and are beyond our control.

This also applies to our health. It is just something that doesn't occur overnight. You have to work on it every day. Think about gravity-- we'll have to walk against it every day of our existence but we are capable of doing this. Same goes for our health. Once we are armed with the necessary means to achieve it, we can easily work towards its achievement.

But there is no point on making it so complex, as many folks many times do. These are just a few queries to raise to yourself to help pave the way for health and rejuvenation.

- How can I enjoy today eating properly and working out?
- What foods can I eat that are healthy and taste delicious?
- What type of exercise or activity can I do that I enjoy doing?
- How can I fuel my system with the foods that it requires?
- Why do I have to eat properly?
- Why should I exercise today?

THE 9 KEY HABITS OF HEALTHY FOLKS

Now that you are familiar with the basic stages of the chiropractic science, we can jump to the 9 essential habits that healthy folks practice on a daily basis which are vital for your health. This information will help you take more thoughtful and life-changing decisions.

These 9 habits trigger substantial lifestyle adjustments, one part a time. Like in the case of every new change, if you push it too aggressively and fast, you will most likely burn out and come up with the excuse later that "it just didn't work out" and quit from making another attempt. In the upcoming chapters, we'll explain these 9 habits in great detail but for the moment, here are the key principles.

1. Water/Hydration

Everyday we'll joyously sip our cup of coffees and sodas. But when it comes to actually drinking glass of water, we just brush it off. We just can't force ourselves to drink it that easy. But drinking plain water is vital for our health--afterall, 95% of our systems are made of water and not coffee or a fizzy drink. Furthermore, water is able to expel toxins from our systems, and various studies have confirmed that drinking at least eight glasses of water daily can yield a substantial impact on the system's power to preserve health and fight of disorders.

2. Veggies

Some may feel like puking whenever they see veggies. But our parents weren't wrong when they told us back when we were kids to eat our veggies, especially green ones that are full of vitamins like spinach and broccoli. Increasing your daily consumption of greens is one of the wisest nutrition decisions you can make for your health. Consider this from a scientific perspective. When greens are out in the nature, they transmute light into energy, a procedure called "photosynthesis". By consuming wholesome and raw green leafy greens, you are taking this energy from the plants. We have stated "raw" here, because we are going to explain the misconception of cooked greens later on.

3. Antioxidant nutrients.

Antioxidants are the key foe of destructive free radicals, which are bad cell reactions raising daily as we age. Excessive free radicals have been connected to cancer in some studies. However, free radicals are not only triggered by the aging process as other factors like stress, injuries, or bad diet rich in processed and chemical loaded foods come into play.

Our parents would always tell us to eat our veggies and fruits and they had a point on doing so. Studies have also validated that our parents advice to eat fruits and veggies really pays off. One of the key factors that makes their consumption healthy, is the fact that they are naturally fortified with antioxidant nutrients. This a broad term with a rather simple explanation. Mary Beth Russell, registered dietician validates that Antioxidants are essentially nutrients that you consumer from your food that ensure the proper function of the cellular reactions that are supposed to happen inside your system.

An abundance of antioxidant substances in your systems, makes it more capable of fighting and eradicating inflammatory diseases like heart problems, diabetes, cataracts, and even cancer. But here is an issue. Only a very small minority of 7% of Americans consume sufficient amounts of antioxidant nutrients daily. This is a bit of surprise as antioxidants are not scarce to find--they are found in fruits, veggies, tea and even wine. As matter of fact, the more vivid color a fruit or veggie has, the more antioxidants they most likely contain. So how many antioxidants should we take on daily basis? Experts say 5 portions of fruits or veggies per day e.g a fruit for breakfast, 1-2 veggies for lunch, 1 fruit or veggie for snack time, and 1 veggie for dinner. This is an easy addition to your diet that will pay off for the years to come.

4. Healthy Oils

Even though we tend to pile on fat inside our bodies to a great degree, we seriously lack enough fatty acids that could benefit our health. Based on studies, the mean person has a lack of vital fatty acids that reaches 90%! Insufficient E.F.A intake is connected with heart and brain problems among a huge range of other inflammatory disorders. Now, that doesn't mean that you have to swallow that bottle of vegetable oil that's stored in your cabinet. Only certain oils are healthy and these are fish oils and flaxseed oils. We are going to elaborate on this further in a later section.

5. Proper oxygenation

It is important to repeatedly allow proper oxygenation of the tissues through mindful breathing methods (here is where cardio exercise can help you out). In reality, every few of us know how to breathe properly. We are going to mention the right techniques of breathing in the next sections.

6. Good Posture

A good reason why we are unable to breath properly, is because we have a wrong posture in the first place. When we stand or sit and squeeze ourselves, we place strain on our breathing canals as well, including our diaphragm and lungs. Bad posture additionally causes other issues. It puts stress in the spinal curve and this causes issues with the nervous system. It can also bear an impact in our moods also, as we'll examine later in this report.

7. Physical activity/exercise

Yep, we know that this is challenging and we all come-up with various excuses not to get ourselves moving. But whether you like it or not, exercise and physical activity in general is vital for your health. There are no excuses such as babysitting, running around doing house chores, or being too busy. What your system needs is a complete cardio workout plan which activates a very vital muscle in your system and that is the heart. You have to challenge it in positive manner to get it moving more blood and oxygen throughout your body. The more you can trigger it, the better it will work for your system.

8. Adequate sleep

It's no surprise that Americans lack sufficient amounts of sleep, every day. We are reportedly so busy being like that, that we neglect the necessity of sleeping adequately every night and complete a full 8 hours of sleep. The issue is, insufficient sleep is a vital culprit of poor health. People who don't sleep enough have a higher risk of suffering from poor immune system capacity. So besides inducing tiredness and fatigue, lack of sleep can also lead to the onset of other issues due to suppressed immunity.

9. Positive mindset

We don't want to sound like we have our head in the clouds or promote new-age stuff, but there is a point in having a positive mindset. If let's say you catch a cold and your mourn and complain about it, you will end up feeling worse. But if you work with it instead of "cursing it' and don't pay much attention, you'll recover faster, almost magically. Of course, this doesn't imply that you should go kickboxing or run a mile when you are ill. This is a signal that maybe your system need some resting time so take a break. But don't focus too much on that or you will feel worse.

By practicing these 9 lifestyle habits and believe in them, you will manifest a more healthy reality for yourself. Towards the next sections, we are going to explain these in more detail.

CHAPTER 6: THE LOW BACK PAIN STATISTICS

What is Backpain?

Back pain is a very common medical problem and affects around 8 out of 10 people during their lives. The back pain intensity varies from dull and constant pain to sudden, sharp pain. Back pain can be acute if it comes on suddenly and lasts only for a few days to a few weeks. It is considered a chronic condition if it lasts for more than a few months.

In the U.S., approximately 16 million adults, which is 8 percent of all adults, experience chronic or persistent back pain. This affects their everyday activities in a certain way.

Causes of Backpain

Back pain is one of the common types of pain among adults in the United States. It can be caused due to multiple reasons, such as strained muscles or ligaments, poor posture, vigorous everyday activities, excess weight, or psychological problems. According to a Statista survey, around 29 percent of U.S. adults with back problems mentioned that stress was the main cause of their pain, while 26 percent mentioned lack of exercise and weak muscles as the cause. The remaining 29 percent blamed physical work.

<u>Muscle or ligament strain</u>:

Strain in the back muscle and spinal ligaments may occur due to a sudden jerk during physical activity or repeated heavy lifting.

<u>Bulging or ruptured disks</u>: The disks present between the vertebrae may press on the nerve after rupture or bulge.

<u>Arthritis</u>: Osteoarthritis is also a cause of lower back pain. In some cases, spinal stenosis, i.e., narrowing of the space between the spinal cord due to arthritis, may cause back pain.

<u>Osteoporosis</u>. The brittle and porous bones in the back is also a common cause of back pain.

Treatment of Back Pain

Physical therapy can be used to strengthen the muscles so that they can support the spine. Physical Therapy also improves flexibility and helps in avoiding any other injury.

Depending on the type of back pain, various medications that a doctor may prescribe are:

Oral Pain relievers:

Nonsteroidal anti-inflammatory drugs (NSAIDs), like ibuprofen and naproxen sodium, can be used to relieve back pain. These medications can be taken as Over-The-Counter Pain killers as well, but taking as per a doctor's prescription is recommended.

Topical pain relievers:

Painkillers in the form of creams, ointments, sprays, or patches help to relieve the pain.

Muscle relaxants:

If painkillers do not provide relief, the doctor may prescribe muscle relaxants.

Narcotics:

Drugs with opioids, such as oxycodone or hydrocodone, can be used for a short time as prescribed by the doctor. Opioids cannot be used for chronic back pain.

Antidepressants:

If stress or depression is the cause, the doctor may prescribe antidepressants, such as duloxetine (Cymbalta), and tricyclic antidepressants, such as amitriptyline. These drugs have been shown to relieve chronic back pain even independently of their effect on depression.

Steroids:

Steroid injections can be used in the treatment of lower back pain. Steroid injections help in reducing inflammation and pain.

Complications associated with the treatment of lower back pain:

If antidepressants are used, they may cause various complications such as arrhythmia, tachycardia, erectile dysfunction, diabetes, and suicidal thoughts. Steroid injections may cause cartilage damage, nerve damage, or joint infection.

Based on traditional medicine, spinal surgery might be considered necessary in the case of a severe compromise of strucutural integrity of which nothing else can remedy. Complications can arise from this type of intervention, such as pneumonia after surgery, deep vein thrombosis, nerve injury, and infection at the surgical site.

Facet syndrome

Every day, a large number of people suffer from backpain. Facet joint syndrome is one of the major causes of back pain but is rarely discussed. Facet syndrome is a spinal disorder that affects the entire spine, from top to bottom, from the neck to the sacrum. Facet joints are found on the sides of the spine and allow the vertebrae to stack up high, resulting in a flexible spine. Facet joints are formed by superior and inferior facets on either side of each vertebra. When combined with the intervertebral disc, these facet joints constitute a tri-complex that allows rotatory motions of the spine, such as bending forward and bending backward.

During backward movements, the back section of the intervertebral disc squishes and forces the facets nearer together. These facet joints can be easily harmed due to the spine's constant wear and tear movements.

Inflammation of the joints and arthritis will result in chronic back pain and muscle spasms. The usual joint capsule will be thinner, and the amount of synovial fluid will be reduced in the inflammatory phase. From a microscopic perspective, the cartilage between the two joints is either thinned out or destroyed in facet joint syndrome.

Facet joint syndrome is prevalent in people over the age of 50. The lifetime adult prevalence of facet syndrome in the USA is approximately 65 - 85%.

Cause of Facet syndrome

The degeneration of the spine, also known as spondylosis, is the most common cause of facet Syndrome.

Obesity or being overweight can result in accelerated deterioration of the facet joints. Poor posture, repeated bending or twisting movements, sedentary lifestyle, abrupt forceful stretching or ligament tear, trauma from accidents, and sports injury will hasten the development of facet arthritis or worsen the symptoms of pre-existing facet arthritis.

Facet syndrome is anatomically distinguished by restricted joint space, uneven bony prominences, and bony spurs (overgrowth of bones in the joint space).

Diagnosis of Facet Syndrome

X-rays, CT scans, and MRIs can be used to assess the vertebral bones and joints. Diagnostic injection tests using anaesthetic or steroids are also used. If the injection relieves the pain, a probable diagnosis is found.

Treatment of Facet Syndrome

Conservative Treatment:

The initial line of treatment for the vast majority of patients is conservative management. Modification of activities, rest, and physical therapy are examples of conservative treatment. Correct posture in standing, sitting, and sleeping positions is essential to reduce the facet syndrome. Without engaging in strenuous activities in the first several weeks, rest is required to enable optimal joint healing.

Physical Medicine the likes of chiropractic is extremely important since stretching and flexibility exercises are recommended long-term to avoid recurrence. These exercises will strengthen the muscles and prevent and eradicate unnecessary joint movements. Weight-bearing on the most vulnerable parts of the body is done by the spine and back muscles, strengthening the back and preventing joint arthritis.

Medications:

Medications such as pain relievers, anti-inflammatory medications, and muscle relaxants are always helpful and are usually prescribed by the doctor to help patients recover from the acute phase.

Other treatment methods:

Lumbar and cervical neck collars for support are beneficial in pain relief. These will support the spine's weight and relieve the load on the spine. The external support benefits the neck and back.

Weight loss is critical in taking stress from the arthritic joints in conservative therapy.

Minimally Invasive Surgery:

When conservative treatment is no longer effective, surgery is unfortunately unavoidable in some cases. In this instance, a needle is inserted into the facet joint to administer the drugs, anaesthetics, and steroids into the joint. This is a minimally invasive surgical technique. This is done as an outpatient procedure involving x-rays to obtain a facet joint's view. When the facet joint cannot be seen, the guidance view through the endoscope is employed in some circumstances.

When injections fail or pains recur, radiofrequency ablation can be recommended. Using **microelectrode heat therapy**, the nerve responsible for pain generation is ablated during this treatment. The microelectrode needle is inserted where the nerve to the joint is passing. The patient will not feel the pain as a result of this. It provides long-term relief from facet joint discomfort. It is used to control the pain over a period of 12 months.

Surgery:

Surgical procedures such as spinal fusion and facet debridement might be used when more permanent remedies are required. Spinal fusion is a more invasive treatment that may result in more complications than the other procedure. It also takes a bit longer to heal. According to studies, the recovery success rate is 66% in spinal fusion.

Complications associated with the treatment of Facet Syndrome:

Conservative therapy provides short-term relief and does not treat the condition. The minimally invasive surgery may cause infection, bleeding, or nerve damage. Local paralysis of limbs or anesthesia may result due to invasive procedures and surgery.

Degenerative Disc Disease

Degenerative disc disease is a condition in which one or more vertebral discs in the spine lose their strength and leads to pressure on the adjacent nerves. It is one of the most common causes of low back and neck pain. It is a progressive condition that occurs over time due to wear and tear or injury. The spinal discs may show signs of wear and tear as we get older and begin to break down; thus, they may not work as well. This condition is very common in old age.

It primarily affects the lower back but might extend to the legs and hips. It worsens due to twisting or bending, or even sitting. Walking and exercise usually help to reduce the pain.

In the U.S., about 40% of adults over the age of 40 have at least one degenerated vertebral disc. By the age of 80, this percentage increases to 80%. The neck (cervical spine) and lower back (lumbar spine) are the most common sites of this condition. It can also cause back pain in about 5% of adults.

Causes of Degenerative Disc Disease:

The wear and tear of the spinal discs is the major cause of this condition. This can occur due to:

Age:

During old age, wear and tear of vertebral discs are common as a physiological change in the body.

Dry out:

The disks in the spine have water. As a person ages, the discs lose water and get thinner. The thin disks can't absorb shocks properly, and this also reduces the cushion or padding between the vertebrae. This can lead to pain. If due to a condition, drying out of the discs occur at a lower age, a similar condition may occur.

Obesity or sedentary lifestyle:

This weakens the muscles and joints and thus, leads to the condition.

Injury:

Injury may cause wear and tear of the disc and thus, cause the condition.

Diagnosis of Degenerative Disc Disease:

X-ray, CT scan or MRI can be used to check the bone, joint, and nerves.

Treatment of Degenerative Disc Disease

Chiropractic:

Decompression therapy, strengthening and stretching exercises with a chiropractor specialized in the treatment of this type of condition can help restore the integrity of the disc, and bring about greater stability to the regions. This in turn, can help better manage the condition.

Medications:

With regards to mainstream medicine, the standard of care unfortunately is to cover up symptoms with medication. This in turn has brought about the opioid epidemic because of the gross negligence of the root cause of the source of the pain. Pain relievers and muscle relaxants are what mainstream pain specialists use to reduce the pain and inflammation and relax the muscles.

Steroid injections:

When pain medication fails, pain specialists often resort to steroid injections near the area of injury helps to attempt to reduce the pain, swelling, and inflammation. A short needle is usually given in the epidural space in the back. This approach usually leads to short term relief, only prolonging the problem and making the issue worse long term.

Radiofrequency neurotomy:

Another somewhat barbaric approach to treating pain is using electric currents to burn sensory nerves in the affected area to prevent pain signals from reaching the brain.

Surgery:

If other treatments do not provide relief, the standard approach would be to just cut out what is wrong, which is insane. When all else fails, cut it out is the motto in healthcare. A type of spinal decompression surgery can be performed.

1. Diskectomy: In this surgery, the injured part of the spinal disc is removed to relieve the pressure on the nerves and other adjacent structures.
2. Foraminotomy: In this surgery, tissue or bone is removed the expand the opening of the affected nerve roots.
3. Spinal fusion: Two or more vertebral bones are connected or fused to improve stability during this procedure.

Complications associated with the treatment:

Steroid injections may cause cartilage damage, nerve damage, or joint infection. At the same time, surgery can lead to various complications such as nerve injury, infection at the surgical site, and rupture of adjacent structures.

Lumbar Arthritis

The spine has five main sections, the cervical, thoracic, lumbar, sacrum, and coccyx. Arthritis in the lumbar region of the spine, known as Lumar arthritis, is another common cause of back pain. Lumbar arthritis or Lumbar spine osteoarthritis affects approximately 30% of males and 28% of females of age 55–64 in the United States. According to a study, over 50 million Americans have a form of doctor-diagnosed arthritis.

Lumbar arthritis or spinal arthritis is not a disease or a condition. Instead, it is a symptom of different forms of arthritis that affect the spine. Osteoarthritis is the most common cause of lumbar arthritis. Lumbar arthritis causes chronic pain or lingering soreness in the lower back. Muscle spasms, reduced range of motions, and creaking sounds from the joints with pain are some other common symptoms.

Causes of Lumbar Arthritis

Spondyloarthritis:

Spondyloarthritis affects the spine and sacroiliac joints, the joints that are located between the sacrum and pelvic bones. This causes inflammation of tendons and ligaments near the joint and thus, leads to lumbar arthritis.

Psoriatic arthritis:

This condition usually affects people with psoriasis. According to the Arthritis Foundation, about 20% of people with psoriatic arthritis have spine involvement. It can also lead to bony overgrowth, causing fusion of the vertebrae. Thus, it can lead to stiffness and pain with movement.

Enteropathic arthritis:

People with inflammatory bowel diseases (Crohn's disease and ulcerative colitis) may have enteropathic arthritis. This can lead to arthritis in the lumbar region of the spine.

Reactive arthritis:

Bacterial infections caused by chlamydia or salmonella can also lead to arthritis in the lumbar region of the spine.

Osteoporosis:

In Osteoporosis, the bone loses it becomes brittle. This brittle bone is prone to injury even due to the minimum traumas. Osteoporosis usually occurs in old age or due to a decrease in hormones and chronic inflammatory diseases. When seen in the spine, the vertebrae bones become weak and brittle. This can become painful with time. This increases the chance of bone fracture in the lumbar region and thus, can lead to lumbar arthritis.

Lumbar Osteoarthritis:

This is seen when the cartilage that protects the lumbar vertebral joints breaks down, exposing small nerves within the bone.

Diagnosis of Lumbar arthritis:

X-rays, CT scans, MRI scans, or bone density studies are helpful to diagnose the condition.

Treatment of Lumbar Arthritis:

Conservative treatment:

According to the AMA, this association recommends the utilization of chiropractic care before surgery. This is a stark contrast to their position merely 40 years ago when they attempted to destroy the chiropractic profession because they considered chiropractors a direct threat to their financial bottom line. Spinal adjustments can be used as first-line therapy for low back pain during lumbar arthritis.

Lifestyle changes such as losing weight, quitting smoking, and taking a healthy diet are helpful in managing the condition and reducing the intensity and symptoms.

Medication:

If non-invasive therapies are not utilized, a medical doctor often recommends painkillers (like acetaminophen), including Over-The-Counter painkillers, can be used to reduce pain and inflammation. Antirheumatic drugs (DMARDs) can be used to reduce the progress of the disease.

Physical therapy:

Weight-bearing exercises are beneficial in increasing the bone mineral density of the lumbar spine. Exercising under the observation of a physical therapist helps provide long-term relief and treat the condition. Aerobics and Yoga are also some of the effective exercises to manage this condition.

Surgery:

If mainstream medicine is the portal of entry to pain management, and the traditional avenues of pain reduction medication does not work, which most of the time it doesn't, surgeries such as joint replacement surgery or joint fusion surgery will be used to treat the condition.

Decompression of the spinal cord to reduce the pressure at the spinal nerves or spinal fusion are also some of the surgical procedures that can mainstream pain management specialists use.

Complications associated with the treatment of lumbar arthritis:

Surgery can cause trauma to the adjacent structures, while uncontrolled or incorrect physical therapy may worsen the condition.

Osteoarthritis

Osteoarthritis is sometimes considered a form of Degenerative joint disease. Osteoarthritis affects around 27 million Americans and the chances of the disease increase with age. Most people over age 60 have some form of osteoarthritis. It may also occur in the 20s and 30s can cause osteoarthritis. The cause of osteoarthritis at a young age can be a joint injury or repetitive joint stress from overuse. Women are more affected than men, especially over 50 years of age (post-menopausal). Osteoarthritis usually affects the joints that bear most of the bodyweight, such as the knee and the feet. Osteoarthritis in the spine is also common. Joint pain, soreness, stiffness in the joints, swelling and bony enlargements are the common symptoms.

Osteoarthritis has two main types:

Primary: This is the common type and is generalized. This type usually affects the fingers, thumbs, spine, hips, knees, and big toes.

Secondary: This type is seen due to a pre-existing joint condition such as repetitive or sports-related trauma or injury, rheumatoid arthritis, gout, infectious arthritis, or a genetic joint disorder, such as Ehlers-Danlos.

Causes of Osteoarthritis:

Osteoarthritis occurs if the cartilage that cushions the joint between the ends of bones gradually deteriorates. If the cartilage wears down completely, it causes inflammation and pain.

Age:

Older age is one of the most common causes.

Obesity:

Increased weight and fat deposits due to obesity increase the load and stress on the weight-bearing joints, such as the pelvis, knees, and spine.

Joint injury:

A major joint injury may cause osteoarthritis in the joint at some point in life. Vigorous, repetitive activity or physically demanding jobs can also increase the risk of injury and, thus, osteoarthritis.

Joint overuse:

Overuse of the joints increases the risk of developing osteoarthritis.

Other joint diseases:

Rheumatoid arthritis, an autoimmune condition, also increases the risk of osteoarthritis.

Diagnosis of Osteoarthritis:

X-rays and MRI scans can be done to check the injury at the joint. Lab tests such as blood tests or joint fluid analysis are also helpful in the diagnosis. Blood tests is helpful in ruling out other diseases such as rheumatoid arthritis. Fluid analysis helps in the assessment of the joint fluid.

Treatment of Osteoarthritis

Medications:

Medications can help relieve pain due to osteoarthritis. Acetaminophen (Tylenol) is helpful for mild to moderate pain in osteoarthritis. Nonsteroidal anti-inflammatory drugs (NSAIDs), including Over-the-counter NSAIDs (ibuprofen and naproxen sodium), also help to relieve osteoarthritis pain. Other painkillers can be used based on the doctor's prescription. Duloxetine (Cymbalta) is an antidepressant and is approved to treat chronic pain due to osteoarthritis.

Chiropractic Therapy:

Chiropractic adjustment and therapies can stabilize the osteoarthritic join and bring about greater strength and biomechanical stability to the region. Exercise such as aerobics improves flexibility, joint stability, and muscle strength. The exercise helps to reduce the pain and disability in osteoarthritis. Vigorous exercise should be avoided.

Hot and cold therapies:

Intermittent hot and cold treatments (such as the application of hot and cold packs) can be used for the temporary relief of stiffness and pain.

Steroid injections:

When all else fails the standard approach can often times invlove injecting the area of inflammation with a steroid to temporarily provide relief. But the root of the problem is still there.

Transcutaneous electrical nerve stimulation (TENS):

In this procedure, a low-voltage electrical current is passed at the site to relieve pain. This can provide short-term relief.

Alternative medicine:

According to some medical research, supplements such as glucosamine and chondroitin may relieve pain in some people with osteoarthritis. Acupuncture is another procedure that is effective in immediately relieving the pain.

Supportive devices:

Crutches, shoe inserts or canes help to stabilize the ligaments and tendons and thus, decrease pain.

Surgery:

Lubrication injections: Injections consisting of hyaluronic acid may help to relieve pain by providing some cushioning in the joint.

Joint replacement: In this surgery, the damaged joint surfaces are replaced with a plastic or metal parts. This procedure often times has serious complications with biomechanical recovery.

Complications associated with the treatment of osteoarthritis:

Surgical treatment increases the risk of various complications such as infections and blood clots. Artificial joints can also wear out or become loose and thus, eventually need to be replaced.

CHAPTER 7: SPINAL DEGENERATION

If you are not a hermit or a burning loner, you probably know someone or many people involved in degenerative joint disease (DJD). Also known as osteoarthritis, about 27 million Americans over the age of 25 have DJD, accounting for about 14 percent of the total population of this age group. (1)

Worse, about 34% of those over 65 have a DJD. And as this is more common among the elderly, we can expect these numbers to continue to rise as the proportion of Americans over 65 grows.

What is degenerative joint disease, and this common form of arthritis can be treated naturally? Let's take a look at how diet and lifestyle can help you manage DJD.

What Is a Degenerative Joint Disease (DJD)?

The degenerative joint disease is a progressive disease that attacks the cartilage of the body, the hard tissue that covers the ends of the bones and joints so that the bones can move. DJD is considered the most common form of arthritis and is the leading cause of adult joint pain, affecting mostly the elderly and slowly getting worse with age.

The terms degenerative arthropathy, degenerative arthritis and osteoarthritis (sometimes referred to as osteoarthritis) are often used interchangeably. Both are essentially the same type of disorder that over time causes cartilage wear (the tissue between the bones) and cause great pain in the bones and joints of the process. Osteoarthritis is the degenerative nature that gets worse over time, and unfortunately, there is no "cure" to prevent progression or reverse the damage done. (2)

It can develop osteoarthritis symptoms throughout the body, in one joint, but usually affects the spine (upper and lower back), neck, hips, knees, and hands (especially the fingertips) and the thumb. The symptoms usually include osteoarthritis / joint degeneration: (3)

- Joint pain that can sometimes get worse and "come and go" in terms of pain
- Stiffness (especially in the morning after getting up)
- To postpone problems that get worse as the disease progresses
- More pain, inflammation, and limitations (some people change quickly, but in most cases, the symptoms start to get worse, especially the joints may not work after exercise but become clearer at any time of the day)
- Difficulty in performing daily tasks such as wrinkles, wear, walking, stretching, squats (especially osteoarthritis in the knees) or certain physical tasks while working (though for some osteoarthritis is relatively mild and the days are quite normal) (4)
- When DJD affects your hips, you may feel pain in the groin, thighs, buttocks or knees.

- When DJD affects your joints, it develops small bony spines in your joints and your fingers can become enlarged, injured, hardened and numb
- DJD in the spine can cause numbness in the neck and a stiff lower back
- You can hear the sound of bones when the disease gets serious
- As a side effect of ongoing pain and mobility/work limitations, depression, sleep disorders, hopelessness, and weight changes can sometimes develop.

Natural Treatment of Degenerative Joint Disease / Osteoarthritis

Although it is not always possible to completely cure a post-development degenerative joint disease, there are many natural treatment options for osteoarthritis that can have a great effect. These include: exercising and staying active, avoiding weight gain and maintaining a healthy weight, taking an anti-inflammatory diet and treating pain through physiotherapy, saunas, massage therapy and oils. Essentially, this all helps to reduce the severity of the symptoms and delay the progression of the disease to prevent more cartilage.

The main objectives of all degenerative diseases/osteoarthritis or arthritis are to relieve inflammation/swelling, to control pain, to improve mobility and joint function, to maintain a healthy weight, to exert less pressure on sensitive joints and to improve vision mood, thereby reducing stress to better manage a degenerative disease.

Stay Active

While most people with osteoarthritis typically have joint pain and limited mobility, many find that they feel better and generally experience fewer symptoms while they are moving. In fact, the sport is considered one of the most important treatments for the degenerative joint disease. As the old saying goes, "Move it or lose it." In other words, the more you strengthen and stretch the parts of your body, the better it will stay intact in old age.

Exercise is important to reduce inflammation, increase flexibility, strengthen muscles (including the heart), increase blood circulation, and maintain a healthy body weight. Helps to keep joints and bones strong and supple, improves cardiovascular health and cardiovascular health, increases joint mobility and improves synovial fluid movement throughout the body. Do not forget the mental benefits of sport. Regular exercise is an effective way to relieve stress, improve mood, control stress hormones such as cortisol, and help you sleep better.

Since each DJD patient differs in terms of physical performance and pain perception, the amount and shape of the prescribed exercises will depend on the specific condition of each person and the stability of the joints. The ideal is a combination of three types of exercises for osteoarthritis: (5)

- Strengthening exercises to improve muscle strength, which supports the affected joints, such as exercises to strengthen the knee
- Aerobic activities to improve blood pressure, circulation and inflammation
- Agility activities to keep your joints flexible and help you feel better about your daily movements

The most beneficial and least painful exercises include walking, swimming, and water aerobics. If your training is painful or more active, your doctor or physiotherapist may recommend safer and more useful exercises. Start slowly and find ways to continue your day by developing your strength and strength.

Reduce Inflammation and Support the Cartilage with a Nutrient-Rich Diet

Research indicates that poor nutrition can increase inflammation and increase enzymes that can destroy collagen and other important proteins in order to maintain healthy tissue. The cartilage contains about 65 to 80% water and the rest consists of three components: collagen, proteoglycans, and chondrocytes.

Collagen is a type of fibrous protein that acts as the body's natural "building blocks" for the skin, tendons, bones, and other connective tissues. Proteoglycans are interwoven with collagen in a mesh-like tissue that absorbs shock and vibration from the cartilage, while chondrocytes primarily produce cartilage and help keep it intact in old age.

Some of the ways in which you can help your body maintain valuable cartilage and reduce inflammation include the use of all types of natural anti-inflammatory foods. These provide essential fatty acids, antioxidants, minerals and vitamins that support the immune system, relieve pain and contribute to the healthy formation of tissue and bone.

Focus your diet as much as possible on these foods:

- Fresh vegetables (all types): Pay attention to the variety and at least four to five servings per day
- Whole fruit pieces (without juice): Three to four servings per day are a good source of income for most people

- Herbs, spices, and teas: turmeric, ginger, basil, oregano, thyme, etc., as well as green tea and organic coffee in moderation
- Probiotic foods: yogurt, kombucha, kvass, kefir or vegetables grown
- Wild fish, uncut eggs, and grass / herbal meat: higher levels of omega-3 and vitamin D than the cultivated varieties and excellent sources of protein, healthy fats and essential nutrients such as zinc and selenium and vitamin B. There is evidence that vitamin D is present in patients with arthritis is. Then, if possible, you should add more raw dairy products. (6)
- healthy fats: grass-fed butter, coconut oil, extra virgin olive oil, nuts/seeds
- old grains and legumes/beans: best in germination and 100% unrefined/whole
- Bone broth: contains collagen and helps to maintain healthy joints
- Limit or eliminate foods that promote inflammation:
- Refined vegetable oils (such as rapeseed oil, corn and soybean oil, rich in omega-6-inflammatory fatty acids)
- Pasteurized dairy products (common allergens) and conventional meat, poultry and eggs, which also contain hormones, antibiotics and omega-6 fatty acids that contribute to inflammation
- Refined carbohydrates and processed cereal products and added sugars (in most prepackaged sandwiches, bread, spices, preserves, cereals, etc.)
- Trans fat / hydrogenated fats (in packaged/processed products and often for frying food)

Maintain a Healthy Body Weight

Overweight already contributes to sensitive joints. (7) Osteoarthritis patients who are overweight should try to achieve a healthy body weight in a realistic manner by using a balanced diet and adding more exercise. This should be seen as a long-term change in lifestyle, not as a very low-calorie fast-food diet that can lead to malnutrition to limit more injuries.

Get Enough Rest / Relaxation

If you do not sleep enough, do not go and relax, joints and muscles, it will be harder to repair while stressing hormones, weight and tend to increase the inflammation. They need to get enough sleep every night (usually seven to nine hours) to relieve stressful joints, maintain hormone balance, balance appetite, and repair damaged tissue. Learn to recognize your body's signals and know when to stop or slow down and take a break so you do not feel anxious, overworked and exhausted.

Control the Pain Naturally

Dealing with pain can be one of the most difficult tasks in the fight against degenerative joint disease because it undermines the quality of life, the ability to do good work, and independence. Many doctors prescribe non-steroidal anti-inflammatory drugs (NSAIDs included) or even surgery to relieve pain when the situation becomes severe enough, but you can also use equally effective pain relief techniques. Some of the most popular complementary therapies and alternatives that fight pain are:

- **Acupuncture:** Studies show that patients who receive acupuncture usually have less pain than patients in control groups. It has been shown that acupuncture relieves the symptoms of back and neck pain, muscle pain and joint stiffness, osteoarthritis and chronic headache. (8)
- **Massage Therapy:** A professional massage can help to improve blood circulation, bring blood to sensitive areas, relax the mind and relieve stress.
- **Foot Reflexology:** For centuries foot reflexology has been used to stimulate the nervous system and help the body with stress, fatigue, pain and emotional problems.
- **Treatments with Infrared Sauna:** Heat and cold (or both together, used at different times) can be helpful in relaxing joints and muscles and reducing swelling or pain. (9) At home, you can use warm towels, ice packs, hot bags or a hot shower to relieve pain. Also consider infrared saunas, a type of sauna that uses heat and light to relax the body, generate heat, spray perspiration, and release stored toxins. It has proven pain-relieving and parasympathetic, helping the body to better manage stress.

What Are The Causes Of Osteoarthritis / DJD?

People with DJD do not maintain enough healthy cartilage as they get older, which means that more moving bones become more painful instead of being blocked by the slippery substance that serves as a buffer between the bones. We need cartilage so that the bone "slides" and absorbs the vibrations or shocks that we experience during our movement.

When the disease has progressed, rub the bones in a manner that causes inflammation, swelling, pain, loss of flexibility and sometimes changes in joint shape.

Here is a brief description of how joints work. The joints are the point where two bones are connected and the shape (in most cases), the following parts: the cartilage, the joint capsule (hard membrane pockets that enclose all the bones), the synovium (inside) capsules) and responsible for the secretion of synovial fluid) and synovial fluid (tampons and lubricates joints and cartilage). (10)

In people with DJD or other forms of joint damage (such as rheumatoid arthritis), their joints are covered with smooth and synovial fluid-coated cartilage, which contributes to the cartilage of the "slide" bone to the bone.

In severe cases of the degenerative joint disease, they begin to shrink and also change shape, while small bone deposits (called osteophytes, sometimes called spurs) can also form on the edges of the joints if they are not. The main problem is that bone spurs can be removed at any time from the cartilage, where they develop and reach the space where the joints are located, causing pain and complications.

Risk Factors for Degenerative Joint Disease

What are the causes of osteoarthritis? It is not complete or unknown at this time, but the disease appears to be caused by a combination of factors that increase a person's risk, including: (11)

- Age (it's more common in people over 65, but anyone can develop DJD) (12)

- To be a woman (it's interesting to note that more men than women have osteoarthritis before the age of 45, but more common in women after 45)
- Overweight or obesity
- Suffer from joint injuries that lead to malformations
- Regular work or hobby that puts great pressure on the joints or requires repeated movements
- Have certain genetic defects that affect the development of cartilage and collagen in the joints
- Have DMD / osteoarthritis in your family (you develop this condition more often if your parents or grandparents have it) (13)

Ask yourself, what is the difference between osteoarthritis and rheumatoid arthritis (RA)? Rheumatoid arthritis is the second most common form of arthritis after arthritis and degenerative arthropathies. RA is considered an autoimmune disease because it attacks the immune system that attacks healthy body tissues that make up the joints. Osteoarthritis is caused by mechanical wear of the joints and is not classified as an autoimmune disease. (14)

DJD and RA produce pain, swelling, arthritis and, over time, joint damage or malformations. Compared to RA, DJD usually starts later in life. Rheumatoid arthritis can occur early in life or middle-aged and usually causes symptoms other than joint/cartilage tissue loss, including fatigue, decreased immunity and sometimes fever, changes in the skin tissue, lungs and eyes or blood vessels.

Key Points of Degenerative Joint Disease:

- Degenerative joint disease, also known as osteoarthritis, is the leading type of arthritis in adults.
- DJD causes a reduction in cartilage and joint tissue that causes joint pain, swelling and movement problems.
- It is caused by a combination of factors: genetics, severe inflammation, poor diet, inactivity, repetitive movements and aging ("normal wear" of the body).

It can help prevent and treat degenerative joint disease in a natural way by taking a nutritious diet, staying active, relieving stress and relieving pain using alternative treatments such as acupuncture, massage, and heat treatments.

CHAPTER 8: THE DANGERS AND RISKS OF ANESTHESIA AND SPINAL SURGERY

Anesthesia is a procedure where a combination of medications are administered to put one in a sleep-like state before major medical procedures, for instance, surgeries. Under anesthesia, one falls in a state of complete unconsciousness and does not feel pain. General anesthesia often uses a combination of inhaled gases and intravenous drugs.

General anesthesia is a very safe procedure; however; it is the surgical procedures that carry the most risks. Some of the examples of these risks include:

i. Obstructive sleep apnea: where one suddenly stops breathing while asleep
ii. Postoperative confusion: this is an acute confusion in the first hours and days following surgery. This condition can occur at any age but is more common in adults (Leslie DL, 2008).
iii. Perioperative Stroke: this is a stroke that occurs within 30 days after surgery. This complication is more common in cardiac, neurologic or vascular procedures (Mashour GA, 2011).

COMPLICATIONS OF SPINAL SURGERY

Most spinal surgeries are performed under general anesthesia. Complications from anesthesia are rare but serious. These complications may be caused by drug reactions stemming from some other medical conditions and include, but not limited to:

i. Bleeding: bleeding may happen when damage is done to major blood vessels following a surgical procedure. It can be very dangerous to a surgical patient.

ii. Blood clotting: following surgeries, and especially major surgeries that require bed rest, blood flow may slow down to the point of causing it to clot. Patients are encouraged to move around as soon as possible after any given surgical procedure to prevent this complication.

iii. Dural tear: dural tears occurs when the thin, protective covering of the spinal cord and spinal nerves is torn, causing several complications including spinal headaches.

iv. Wound infections: the risk of infections following surgical operation is small in most patients, provided proper wound care and hygiene are practiced. However, if an infection does develop, it may be superficial at the level of the skin incision, or it can spread to deeper structures, for example around the vertebrae and the spinal cord in back surgeries.

v. Lung infections: Also known as pneumonia, lung infections may occur after spine surgeries due to prolonged bed rest, viruses or bacteria.

vi. Kidney damage: the possibility of one's kidney getting damaged during surgical operation is almost certain. Protective measures, therefore, must be made to minimize this risk.

vii. Death: there is always a risk of death, especially with major surgical operations.

These complications that occur from spinal surgeries may impact treatment outcomes, leading to the need for further surgical procedures. In addition to alternative surgical procedures, key preventive measures ought to be taken in consideration to avoid serious consequences.

INEFFECTIVENESS OF OTHER JOINT SURGERIES

As with most surgical procedures, carpal tunnel release is not without its risks. In some cases of carpal tunnel release, general anesthesia is used. This is done to put patients into deep sleep during surgery. However, anesthesia poses risks to carpal tunnel release surgeries, which include:

i. Bleeding
ii. Infection
iii. Injury to the median nerve or nerves
iv. Injuries to nearby blood vessels

The recovery from carpal tunnel surgery takes time – anywhere from several weeks to several months. Recovery may take longer if nerves suffered from compression for a long period of time. Recovery involves splinting your wrist and getting physical therapy to strengthen the wrist and hand and promote healing. There may be other risks, depending on your specific medical condition. Be sure to discuss any concerns with your doctor before the procedure.

Strengthening muscles in exercise therapy groups is done in hopes to counteract osteoarthritis, a type of arthritis that often occurs in patients who have undergone surgery for a meniscus injury.

In principle, there are two different types of meniscus injury:

i. Acute injuries - which often occur in young people who might, for example, twist a knee, and;
ii. Wear and tear injuries - which are the first sign that the joint is beginning to break down. This is also referred to as Osteoarthritis.

Young people with acute injuries should undergo surgery. That way, the meniscus can continue to protect the cartilage in the joint. Damage due to wear and tear cannot be repaired surgically, but the joint can be cleared of worn tissue that would otherwise cause the knee to lock or give way.

POSSIBILITIES OF OPIOID USE POST SURGERY

Opioids are drugs which are derived from opium and include several members, such as morphine. Opioids are synthetic and semi-synthetic drugs such as fentanyl, hydrocodone and oxycodone (Offermanns, 2008). They help in reducing pain after surgical procedures by binding to opioid receptors which are found mainly in the peripheral and the central nervous system and the gastrointestinal tract.

Opioids, like other drugs, have side effects which may include itchiness, nausea, euphoria, respiratory depression, sedation and constipation. On the long run, the use of opioids can cause tolerance, which means that increased doses are needed to achieve the same effect, and physical dependence, meaning that the body would depend on doses of opioids to function normally. Furthermore, physical dependance leads to unpleasant withdrawal symptoms upon abrupt discontinuation of the drug (Cicero TJ, 2017). Despite these adverse effects, opioids are of great importance after a surgical procedure, especially for the following medical uses:

i. Acute pain: opioids are efficient in controlling acute pain. For the immediate relief of moderate to acute pain, opioids are frequently the treatment of choice because of their rapid onset, lower risk of dependence and efficacy (Alexander GC, 2012). Additionally, opioids are vital in palliative care to help with controlling severe, chronic, and disabling pain that may occur in some terminal conditions such as cancer.

ii. Diarrhea and constipation: opioids are used in cases of diarrhea-predominant irritable bowel syndrome to suppress bowel movements. On the other hand, the ability to suppress diarrhea may lead to constipation when opioids are used beyond the recommended dose. A remedy to this has been however advanced.

iii. Shortness of breath: opioids help with symptoms of shortness of breath specifically in terminal patients suffering from advanced diseases such as cancer.

Based on the adverse effects and medical uses of opioids as highlighted above, the possibilities of them being used are much higher and should therefore be encouraged. This is because they will prevent costly and more severe complications such as cancer.

THE PREVALENT RISKS OF SURGERY

Basically, the prevalence of risks associated with surgical procedures can be alarming for some people. These risks generally include the following:

i. Collapsed lung: The kidneys are found close to the lung. Thus, the space around the lung may be inadvertently opened during surgical procedure. If this occurs, the lung may collapse due to the difference in pressure between the chest cavity and the outside air.
ii. Urinary tract infection: this can be an infection of the kidneys or the urinary bladder.
iii. Shock: this is a severe drop in the blood pressure that causes a dangerous slowing of the flow of blood throughout the body. It may be caused by the loss of blood, injuries to the spine, infection and metabolic disturbances.
iv. Deep vein thrombosis: this is a blood clot in a large vein deep inside an arm, leg or any other part of the body.
v. Pulmonary embolism: this serious condition occurs when a blood clot breaks away from the vein it was found inside and travels to the lungs. In the lungs, this clot can completely cut off the flow of blood, which is why pulmonary embolism is a medical emergency that causes death in postoperative patients.
vi. Death: whether due to surgeries or post-surgical complications, death is always a risk that exists with any major operation.

EFFECTS AND DANGERS OF OTC DRUGS

Over the counter (OTC) drugs are those drugs that one can buy from stores without a doctor's prescription. They help treat, manage, or prevent common health problems such as allergies, constipation, cold and nausea.

At times, OTC drugs may cause adverse effects. Adverse effects are those that the OTC drugs have on your body but are not intended as part of the action of the OTC drug, or do not help in treating your symptoms. Most of them are unpleasant, like nausea, dizziness or bleeding in the digestive tract. Adverse effects may also include:

i. Drug-food interactions: Food may change how your body processes some OTC drugs, which may prevent them from working the way they should.

ii. Allergic reactions: this is when one's body is allergic to certain medicines or some of the components of OTC drugs.

iii. Drug-drug interactions: our bodies process every medicine differently. When medicines are used together, the ways they affect the body can change. It can increase the chances that one may have side effects from medicines that they are taking. The main interaction types are:

   a. Opposition; Medicines with active ingredients that have opposite effects on one's body this may reduce the effectiveness of one.

   b. Duplication; this is taking two medicines that have similar active ingredients. Too much of this can hurt one's kidney or liver

CHAPTER 9: THE DANGERS OF CORTICOSTEROID INJECTIONS

Corticosteroids are human-made drugs that closely resemble cortisol, a hormone that your adrenal glands produce naturally. Corticosteroids are often referred to by the shortened term "steroids." Corticosteroids are different from the male hormone-related steroid compounds that some athletes abuse. Corticosteroids are medications that mimic the effects of the hormone cortisol, which is produced naturally by the adrenal glands. Cortisol affects many parts of the body, including the immune system. It helps lower levels of prostaglandins and downplays the interaction between specific white blood cells (T-cells and B-cells) involved in the immune response. Corticosteroids stimulate this effect to control inflammation.

They are powerful medications used in short-term and long-term treatment of many conditions. They are used systemically, topically and locally. Systemic use is by either ingesting the medication orally or having it injected intravenously or less commonly by intramuscular injection. Topically is when the drug is used as a cream, ointment or lotion, or is inhaled or used as a nasal spray to treat lung or nasal conditions. Local use is when the medication is injected directly into or near the area it is needed, like in tendonitis or bursitis as well as in epidural injections for back or neck problems.

Corticosteroids are used to provide relief for inflamed areas of the body. They lessen swelling, redness, itching, and allergic reactions. They are often used as part of the treatment for a number of different diseases, such as severe allergies or skin problems, asthma, or arthritis. Corticosteroids may also be used for other conditions as determined by your doctor.

Corticosteroids are powerful medicines. In addition to their helpful effects in treating your medical problem, they have side effects that can be very serious. If your adrenal glands are not producing enough cortisone-like hormones, taking this medicine is not likely to cause problems unless you take too much of it. If you are taking this medicine to treat another medical problem, be sure that you discuss the risks and benefits of this medicine with your doctor.

Why Are They Used To Reduce Pain In An Area Of The Body?

The human body naturally produces cortisol (and other hormones) from the adrenal glands which reside above the kidneys. Corticosteroids mimic these hormones' effects on the body, and when prescribed in a high enough dosage, they suppress the immune system, resulting in decreased overall inflammation levels in the patient.

Cortisone injections are given to a patient to help ease the pain or relieve the inflammation in a particular part of the body. They are generally injected in the joints - ankle, knee, hip, elbow, shoulder, wrist, and even the spine. A cortisone injection is administered for treatment of a variety of conditions. Some of the more commonly known conditions among these include lupus, osteoarthritis, rheumatoid arthritis, gout, and frozen shoulder.

Corticosteroids are medications often used to treat arthritis and related conditions. These medications are widely used because of their overall effectiveness in reducing inflammation--the process that causes the joint pain warmth and swelling of arthritis and related conditions. Examples of corticosteroids include cortisone prednisone and methylprednisolone. These medications are related to cortisol which occurs naturally in the body. Cortisol is a hormone that controls many essential body functions. You could not live without cortisol.

They are commonly used in the practice of pain management for their anti-inflammatory properties. These agents, produced by the adrenal cortex, are widely used in epidural, joint, peripheral nerve and various types of soft tissue injections. Corticosteroids can be classified as an anti-inflammatory (glucocorticoids), androgenic/estrogenic and salt-retaining (mineralocorticoids). Despite these individual classifications, most corticosteroids have some overlapping properties with predictable adverse reactions.

Corticosteroids prescribed to RA patients reduce the levels of inflammation that cause joint pain, stiffness, and bone and cartilage deterioration. Corticosteroids also act as immune system inhibitors (or immune modulators) by suppressing antibody formation and subsequent attacks which cause inflammation in RA patients. Besides RA, corticosteroids are used to treat a number of other inflammatory and autoimmune diseases such as lupus, asthma, skin conditions, and a variety of allergies.

Corticosteroids can be used to treat pain that results from inflammation or edema, which may be cancer-related or non-cancer related. Non-cancer forms of pain that may be treated with corticosteroids include some forms of arthritis including rheumatoid arthritis, ankylosing spondylitis, osteoarthritis, and many others. Treatment may be in the form of tablets or injections directly into joints or soft tissues.

When Were They First Used?

Corticosteroid was first identified by the American chemists Edward Calvin Kendall and Harold L. Mason while researching at the Mayo Clinic. In 1929, Philip S. Hench and colleagues discovered that cortisone is effective in the treatment of rheumatoid arthritis. Kendall was awarded the 1950 Nobel Prize for Physiology or Medicine along with Philip S. Hench and Tadeus Reichstein for the discovery of adrenal cortex hormones, their structures, and their functions. As it turns out, both Reichstein and the team of O. Wintersteiner and J. Pfiffner had separately isolated the compound before Mason and Kendall but failed to recognize its biological significance.

Cortisone was first produced commercially by Merck & Co. in 1948/1949. On September 30, 1949, Percy Julian announced an improvement in the process of producing cortisone from bile acids. This eliminated the need to use osmium tetroxide, a rare, expensive, and dangerous chemical. In the UK in the early 1950s, John Cornforth and Kenneth Callow at the National Institute for Medical Research collaborated with Glaxo to produce cortisone from hecogenin from sisal plants.

Who Discovered These Class Of Medications?

Corticosteroids often called "steroids" were once thought to be miraculous. In 1948, at the Mayo Clinic in Rochester, Minnesota, a group of arthritis patients was given daily injections of a corticosteroid. By the late 1940s, it became clear that to bring autoimmune diseases under good control, it was necessary to suppress inflammation and the immune system. In 1948, E. C. Kendall and P.S. Hench discovered a compound that was miraculously able to suppress inflammation and reverse the symptoms of rheumatoid arthritis. The active component they discovered was a form of corticosteroids.

It all began in September 1948, when a middle-aged woman with rheumatoid arthritis (RA), experiencing severe pain and joint swelling, was first experimentally given a series of corticosteroid injections throughout a few weeks. After the trial period, the woman's symptoms had disappeared, and she got up and walked away from the bed in which she had been confined to for several years. This startling result stunned people throughout the world, and in 1950, P. S. Hench and E. C. Kendall were awarded the Nobel Prize in Physiology and Medicine. It seemed a cure for arthritis had been discovered: corticosteroids.

Philip Hench, Edward Kendall, and Tadeus Reichstein received the Nobel Prize in medicine and physiology in 1950 for their "investigations of the hormones of the adrenal cortex." Hench and Kendall took compound E from the laboratory to the clinic to the Nobel Prize in 2 years.

In 1952, D.H. Peterson and H.C. Murray of Upjohn developed a process that used Rhizopus mold to oxidize progesterone into a compound that was readily converted to cortisone. The ability to cheaply synthesize large quantities of cortisone from the diosgenin in yams resulted in a rapid drop in price to $6 per gram, falling to $0.46 per gram by 1980. Percy Julian's research also aided progress in the field. The exact nature of cortisone's anti-inflammatory action remained a mystery for years after, however, until the leukocyte adhesion cascade and the role of phospholipase A2 in the production of prostaglandins and leukotrienes was fully understood in the early 1980s.

What Is The Mechanism Of How It Works?

Cortisone, a glucocorticoid, and adrenaline are the main hormones released by the body as a reaction to stress. They elevate blood pressure and prepare the body for a fight or flight response. Corticosteroids are typically taken in conjunction with Disease-Modulating Anti-Rheumatic Drugs (DMARDs). For most patients, DMARDs can take weeks to begin working. In this time, it's important to try and get the disease under control as much as possible. Using corticosteroids during this waiting period is a highly effective method of reducing inflammation and helping alleviate pain and stiffness for the patient.

A cortisone injection can be used to give short-term pain relief and reduce the swelling from inflammation of a joint, tendon, or bursa in, for example, the joints of the knee, elbow, and shoulder and into a broken coccyx. Cortisone may also be used to deliberately suppress the immune response in persons with autoimmune diseases or following an organ transplant to prevent transplant rejection. The suppression of the immune system may also be important in the treatment of inflammatory conditions.

Corticosteroids are widely used in the treatment of allergic and inflammatory conditions. It is important to recognize that there are great species differences in the responses to glucocorticoids and that man is a "steroid-resistant" species. Steroids affect metabolism and distribution of T and B lymphocytes, but do not significantly affect antibody production in man. Steroids profoundly affect the inflammatory response by way of vasoconstriction, decreased chemotaxis, and interference with macrophages.

Corticosteroids may also be prescribed during periods of flare-ups, whereby the disease becomes highly active and severe symptoms appear. Corticosteroids are used to quiet down the symptoms and provide immediate relief for patients.

What Are The Short-Term Side Effects With This Type Of Treatment?

In general, corticosteroids are viewed as a "bridge therapy" option for treating RA patients. This means that they are used in select cases for a short period at smaller doses. This is primarily due to the number of severe side effects associated with corticosteroid use.

One of the most common complaints that accompany these cortisone shots is the considerable level of risks involved. Some of the side effects of getting a cortisone injection involve nerve damage, infection of the joint, and the thinning out or death of an adjacent bone. In most cases, the skin and the soft tissue in around the site of the injection thin down. Sometimes, the skin may lighten in complexion, or take on a lighter hue. The tendons around the area may weaken or rupture, and the joint may suffer from temporary pain and inflammation. It is one of the essential things to remember.

Corticosteroids may cause a range of side effects. But they may also relieve the inflammation, pain, and discomfort of many different diseases and conditions. If you work with your doctor to make choices that minimize side effects, you may achieve significant benefits with a reduced risk of such problems.

Because cortisone injections may result in some or all of the side effects mentioned above, the medical community restricts the number of shots that can be injected into a joint. On an average basis, two consecutive cortisone injections must be spaced at least six weeks apart. Also, there must not be more than three to four shots administered on a patient throughout a year.

What Is The Mechanism Of How It Creates This Short-Term Side Negative Side Effect?

Corticosteroids are considered preferred therapy in the treatment of severe acute asthma exacerbations and chronic persistent asthma. Although most asthmatic patients will respond to corticosteroids, there are distinct features of the disease that can make the response to corticosteroids limited or unsustainable.

The adverse effects related to corticosteroids are dose and duration dependent; at conventional doses, they are preventable and easy to monitor. Corticosteroids may cause a range of side effects. But they may also relieve the inflammation, pain, and discomfort of many different diseases and conditions. If you work with your doctor to make choices that minimize side effects, you may achieve significant benefits with a reduced risk of such problems.

For instance, oral use of cortisone has a number of potential systemic side-effects: Asthma, hyperglycemia, insulin resistance, diabetes mellitus, osteoporosis, anxiety, depression, amenorrhoea, cataracts, Cushing's syndrome, and glaucoma, among other problems. Local side effects are rare but can include: pain, infection, skin pigment changes, loss of fatty tissue, and tendon rupture.

Also, injected corticosteroids can cause temporary side effects near the site of the injection, including skin thinning, loss of color in the skin, and intense pain — also known as a post-injection flare. Other signs and symptoms may include facial flushing, insomnia and high blood sugar. Doctors usually limit corticosteroid injections to three or four a year, depending on each patient's situation.

To get the most benefit from corticosteroid medications with the least amount of risk: Try lower doses or intermittent dosing. Newer forms of corticosteroids come in various strengths and lengths of action. Ask your doctor about using low-dose, short-term medications or taking oral corticosteroids every other day instead of daily.

Switch to non-oral forms of corticosteroids. Inhaled corticosteroids for asthma, for example, reach lung surfaces directly, reducing the rest of your body's exposure to them and leading to fewer side effects.

Make healthy choices during therapy. When you're taking corticosteroid medications for a long time, talk with your doctor about ways to minimize side effects. Eat a healthy diet and participate in activities that help you maintain a healthy weight and strengthen bones and muscles.

What Are The Long-Term Side Effects Of This Type Of Treatment?

Corticosteroids are synthetic analogs of human hormones usually produced by the adrenal cortex. They have both glucocorticoid and mineralocorticoid properties. The glucocorticoid components are anti-inflammatory, immunosuppressive, anti-proliferative and vasoconstrictive. They influence the metabolism of carbohydrate and protein, in addition to playing a vital role in the body's stress response.

Mineralocorticoid's main significance is in the balance of salt and water concentrations. Due to the combination of these effects, corticosteroids can cause many adverse effects.

Some of the long-term side effects of corticosteroids include ulcers/gastrointestinal bleeding, osteoporosis, increase the risk of heart disease, decrease in bone density, increased risk of infections, thin skin, bruise easily, slower healing of wounds

Also, steroids that are injected into muscles and joints may cause some pain and swelling at the site of the injection. However, this should pass within a few days. Steroid injections can also cause muscle or tendon weakness, so you may be advised to rest the treated area for a few days after the injection. Other possible side effects can include infections, blushing, and thinning and lightening of the skin in the area where the injection is given. Because of the risk of side effects, steroid injections are often only given at intervals of at least 6 weeks, and a maximum of 3 injections into one area is usually recommended.

Because of the wide variety of medical conditions that corticosteroids treat, it is very important that any conversations with your medical provider include understanding the long-term effects. These effects, both positive and negative, have long-lasting repercussions on our quality of life.

What Is The Mechanism Of How This Treatment Creates This Long-Term Side Effect?

Corticosteroids are powerful medications used in short-term and long-term treatment of many conditions. They are used systemically, topically and locally. Systemic use is by either ingesting the medication orally or having it injected intravenously or less commonly by intramuscular injection. Topically is when the drug is used as a cream, ointment or lotion, or is inhaled or used as a nasal spray to treat lung or nasal conditions. Local use is when the medication is injected directly into or near the area it is needed, like in tendonitis or bursitis as well as in epidural injections for back or neck problems.

Some patients are poor candidates for corticosteroid systemic or locally injected corticosteroid therapy because of conditions that may be made worse by the drugs.

These drugs are called glucocorticoids because of their effect on blood sugar. Use of systemic or locally injected glucocorticoids like prednisone causes a rise in blood sugar levels. This can be in patients with known diabetes or patients with pre-diabetes. It is not uncommon in hospitalized patients to find quite high blood sugars in people not previously diagnosed with diabetes when they are getting high dose prednisone as therapy. This can sometimes require insulin therapy. In general, physicians tend to try to avoid the systemic use of glucocorticoids in patients with diabetes.

Corticosteroids can be used to induce remission or reduce the morbidity in autoimmune diseases. Although high doses can be given for short periods, the aim is to achieve specific targets with the minimum effective dose. Patients who require long-term treatment should be advised about the adverse effects of corticosteroids, particularly the risk of adrenal insufficiency, osteoporosis, and cataracts.

Why Is There A Limit To How Many Injections You Can Receive Per Year Of This Type Of Treatment?

Cortisone injections are commonly used by orthopedic surgeons and other doctors as a treatment for inflammation. While cortisone can be an effective treatment, many doctors will advise against too many cortisone shots. How much is too much, and why do doctors advise against more of something that is seemingly helpful?

Cortisone injections are used in treating multiple common orthopedic conditions, including bursitis, tendonitis, trigger finger, carpal tunnel syndrome, tennis elbow, knee arthritis, and many other overuse conditions. They work by decreasing inflammation of irritated tissues. By limiting the inflammation, pain from these conditions is often relieved.

You should understand that there are reasons not to use cortisone injections, even if they may help some symptoms. Because of this, most orthopedic surgeons will limit the number of cortisone injections they will offer. No more than three cortisone shots in the space of a year is a typical number that many orthopedic surgeons use.

There is no hard and fast rule that says how many cortisone injections can be given over time. However, cortisone injections can have side effects, and repeated use of cortisone injections should be done with caution. Most orthopedic surgeons will choose a number, and advise patients not to exceed that amount of cortisone.

What Does Research Say Overall About The Long-Term Use Of This Type Of Treatment?

The fact that new research is pouring in on the detrimental effects of cortisone injections should not convince anyone that suddenly medicine is being alerted to the risk of corticosteroids. The dangers of cortisone injections have long been known. But in eagerness by health professionals and the patients themselves to get instant relief, the dangers were accepted as part of the treatment, the let's manage the pain until the patient is ready for joint replacement treatment.

Studies on corticosteroids tend to lean toward the extreme use, rather than the average user. For example, some studies look at corticosteroids for extreme and rarer cases of eczema. This makes it harder to research what long-term studies are out there on steroid use. To complicate things further, corticosteroids can be oral, topical, injected, or inhaled, and this dramatically changes the benefits and risks, and in turn the short-term and long-term effects.

Recent research says cortisone may hinder the native stem cells in cartilage. Cortisone threatens their innate regenerative capacity in exchange for temporary analgesia. Corticosteroid injections have been shown to be effective in decreasing the inflammation and pain of ligament injuries for up to 8 weeks; however, these same properties lead to the destruction of cartilage. Simply, the body heals via inflammation; cortisone inhibits inflammation and healing by disrupting the three characteristic phases: inflammatory, proliferative and remodeling.

Finally, the idea that cortisone can cause damage was not an easy sell for some researchers. Corticosteroid injections have been used for a very long time. Their anti-inflammatory and pain relief properties made its use a common practice within the medical community.

CHAPTER 10: STATIN MEDICATIONS AND THEIR CONNECTION TO BACK PAIN

Myth – Cholesterol is Dangerous

Statins are commonly prescribed drugs used to treat high cholesterol. They work by blocking the enzyme that makes cholesterol in the body. Often people treated with statins respond well, and their cholesterol levels lower. In other instances, a person can develop statin intolerance, which can be dangerous. Statin medications lower cholesterol levels in your blood. This can reduce the chance of a heart attack, stroke, and premature death in people who have an elevated risk of developing heart disease or who already have it.

Within the category of anti-lipedimcs there are seven popular statin drugs, but they're not all the same. Some statins are backed by stronger evidence than others that they lower cholesterol or reduce the risk of a heart attack or premature death from heart disease or a stroke. Statin drugs are relatively new, but their use is expanding at a very rapid rate. Some of the most popular statin drugs are zocor, mevacor, lipitor, crestor and several others. These drugs are used to lower or slow down LDL-cholesterol (bad cholesterol) production.

Additionally, along with preventing the production of cholesterol, it is believed to help the body reabsorb that which has already built up as plaque on the walls of arteries. This will help with blood flow but also lessen the chance of this plaque being dislodged and lead to heart attack, stroke and other organ failures.

Statin drugs are extremely dangerous for people with the severe cardiovascular disease. Many studies have shown that the side effects caused by statin medication are far worse than the high cholesterol itself. Medical professionals that claim that these drugs are safe are causing severe damage to the overall health of thousands of people every year.

Why Are They Prescribed?

The class of drugs, called statins, has been a great help to people who need to lower their cholesterol levels. Available by prescription only, these drugs do a wonderful job of lowering cholesterol levels and thereby reducing that person's risk of stroke or heart attack. This class of medication has proven to be so successful that medical professionals estimate that up to 20 million people who are not now on a prescription statin drug would benefit from taking them because of their risk factors for cardiovascular disease.

Statin drugs are currently prescribed like candy for tens of millions of Americans, but you must seriously rethink statin therapy before deciding to take your doctor up on this prescription, as their use has severe and significant consequential side effects and risks, and, their use is clearly not appropriate for everyone.

The majority of people using statin cholesterol-lowering drugs do so as they believe that lowering their cholesterol will prevent heart attacks and strokes. How many of these individuals do you think would continue to take these drugs if they knew that their drugs had been linked to increased risk of heart attack and increased risk of stroke? Probably no one.

With so many side effects of statin drugs, you have to exercise the utmost prudence in opting for the drug. After taking into consideration various factors that adversely affect your overall health, your doctor has to be very careful while prescribing these drugs. Statin alternatives have to be explored with the same diligence.

What Is The Most Common Drug Prescribed For Lowering Cholesterol?

One of the most common drugs prescribed for lowering cholesterol is the statin drug. The statin drug work by blocking a liver enzyme needed to make cholesterol. The body needs some cholesterol to maintain good health. High blood levels of LDL cholesterol and low levels of HDL cholesterol are associated with an increased risk of arterial blockage throughout the body, which could eventually lead to heart attack, stroke, and peripheral artery disease in the legs. Statins may also moderately reduce triglyceride levels, decrease inflammation in arteries, and help raise HDL levels.

Statins are used to reduce cholesterol levels in your body and has become the norm in present-day medicine. Though it is a well-known fact that statin medication gives rise to so many adverse side effects, prescribing this dangerous drug is being projected as the only way to bring down your cholesterol numbers.

In fact, a cholesterol level of 200 is not very dangerous to your health. It can cause serious health implications only when it rises above 400. But modern health professionals blindly make you a "good" candidate for statin drugs as soon as your cholesterol level goes above 200.

Your baseline cholesterol level is tied to the genetic structure of your body. This, of course, varies widely from person to person. Often, this is not taken into account before prescribing statin medication. Your elevated cholesterol may be easily controlled by putting you on a low glycemic diet. This combined with a hormone optimization process can bring down your triglyceride levels. You can totally avoid statin drugs by engaging in regular exercise and adding more fiber to your diet.

What Are Some Of The Symptoms Associated With These Statin Lowering Medications?

Statin intolerance occurs when a person develops side effects from statin use. There are different symptoms you may experience. The most common is muscle pains or cramps, also called myalgias. You may experience muscle inflammation and an elevated marker of muscle injury called creatine kinase. You may experience these symptoms or similar ones while taking statins. These symptoms may not be a result of the medication, but your doctor will conduct tests and get background information to find out.

Statins can also cause liver and muscle toxicity. In severe cases, people have developed rhabdomyolysis. This is a rare condition where muscle cells break down in the body. It causes severe muscle aches and weakness through your entire body. It also causes dark or cola-colored urine. This condition can lead to liver damage and death If not treated.

Statins are safe and well tolerated; however, side effects may occur. They include muscle pain or soreness, leg pain, muscle weakness, generalized pain and weakness, Vomiting, Stomach cramps and Brown discolored urine caused by breakdown of muscles cells being passed in the urine

These symptoms may suggest possible muscle problems such as myopathy and rhabdomyolysis. Rhabdomyolysis is a situation in which the muscle cells break down and cause kidney failure. These symptoms may present a medical emergency and should not be ignored. You should stop taking the statin medication and contact your health-care professional immediately for advice. Liver inflammation may occur with statin use, and often blood tests monitoring liver function are done on a routine basis.

What Does The Research Really Show About What The Effects Are Of Lowering Your Cholesterol?

Cholesterol has been unfairly blamed for just about every case of heart disease for the last 20 years when in reality, you need cholesterol to be healthy; your body uses cholesterol for cell membranes, hormones, neurotransmitters and overall nerve function

Cholesterol is a waxy substance found in your blood and your cells. Your liver makes most of the cholesterol in your body. The rest comes from foods you eat. Cholesterol travels in your blood bundled up in packets called lipoproteins. Cholesterol is not bad for you. The body produces it naturally. But when the body gets too much cholesterol from your diet it becomes dangerous. There are no longer specific levels of "good" and "bad" cholesterol that everyone should have to be considered healthy.

Cholesterol is critical to the normal function of every cell in the body. However, it also contributes to the development of atherosclerosis, a condition in which cholesterol-containing plaques form within arteries. These plaques block the arteries and reduce the flow of blood to the tissues the arteries supply. When plaques rupture, a blood clot forms on the plaque, thereby further blocking the artery and reducing the flow of blood. When blood flow is reduced sufficiently in the arteries that supply blood to the heart, the result is angina (chest pain) or a heart attack. If the reduced flow is caused by plaques in the arteries of the brain, the result is a stroke. If the reduced flow is caused by plaques in the arteries of the leg, they cause intermittent claudication (pain in the legs while walking). By reducing the production of cholesterol, statins can slow the formation of new plaques and occasionally can reduce the size of plaques that already exist. In addition, through mechanisms that are not well understood, statins may also stabilize plaques and make them less prone to rupturing and develop clots.

The real question, however, is why you would want to do that? Lowering cholesterol, the "hype" of the millennium, makes it seem as though you are deriving benefit from the drug therapy and thus improving your overall health. Further, as your health deteriorates from the drugs, other problems which manifest later in life are often misinterpreted as being separate and distinct disorders brought on for alternative reasons rather than associated with the statin use which was truly responsible.

Until recently, statin use has been accepted based on studies which were arranged by the drug company selling the drugs. However, recently these drugs are falling under increased scrutiny. A recent study in Clinical Cardiology found that heart muscle function was "significantly better" in the control group than in those taking statin drugs. Weakened heart muscle function is associated with heart failure.

Is Cholesterol The Real Problem Or Is It Really Inflammation?

Inflammation has become a bit of a buzzword in the medical field because it has been linked to so many different diseases. And one of those diseases is heart disease; the same heart disease that cholesterol is often blamed for. What am I getting at? Well, first consider the role of inflammation in your body. In many respects, it's a good thing as it's your body's natural response to invaders it perceives as threats. If you get a cut, for instance, the process of inflammation is what allows you to heal.

Specifically during inflammation:

- Your blood vessels constrict to keep you from bleeding to death
- Your blood becomes thicker so it can clot
- Your immune system sends cells and chemicals to fight viruses, bacteria and other "bad guys" that could infect the area
- Cells multiply to repair the damage

Ultimately, the cut is healed, and a protective scar may form over the area. If your arteries are damaged, a very similar process occurs inside of your body, except that a "scar" in your artery is known as plaque. This plaque, along with the thickening of your blood and constricting of your blood vessels. Which occur during the inflammatory process, can indeed increase your risk of high blood pressure and heart attacks. Notice that cholesterol has yet to enter the picture. Cholesterol comes in because, to replace your damaged cells, it is necessary.

Remember that no cell can form without it. So if you have a bunch of damaged cells that need to be replaced, your liver will be notified to make more cholesterol and release it into your bloodstream. This is a deliberate process that takes place in your body to produce new, healthy cells. It's also possible, and quite common, for damage to occur in your body on a regular basis. In this case, you will be in a dangerous state of chronic inflammation. The test usually used to determine if you have chronic inflammation is a C-reactive protein (CRP) blood test. CRP level is used as a marker of inflammation in your arteries.

Researchers have identified cholesterols partner in crime as inflammation the flood of white blood cells and chemicals that our immune system unleashes to ward off damage or infection. Cholesterol wouldn't be nearly as dangerous without this process, which is thought to play an essential role in atherosclerosis, the hardening that occurs when low-density lipoprotein (LDL), also known as bad cholesterol, builds up in the arteries.

When high levels of cholesterol occur in the bloodstream, excess LDL begins to seep into the inner wall of the artery. This triggers an inflammatory response, which speeds up the accumulation of cholesterol in the artery wall. This, in turn, produces more inflammation and on and on. Eventually, the deposited cholesterol hardens into a plaque, which can rupture and lead to the blood clots that cause heart attacks and strokes an event that inflammation also appears to help along.

Also, the important role of cholesterol in atherosclerosis is widely accepted by scientists. Research shows that aggressive cholesterol reduction is more beneficial than modest reductions. Nevertheless, atherosclerosis is a complex process that involves more than just cholesterol. For example, scientists have discovered that inflammation in the walls of the arteries may be an important factor in the development of atherosclerosis. In addition to lowering cholesterol levels, statins also reduce inflammation, which could be another mechanism by which statins beneficially affect atherosclerosis. This reduction of inflammation does not depend on statins' ability to reduce cholesterol. Furthermore, these anti-inflammatory effects can be seen as early as two weeks after starting statins.

As A Chiropractor, How Does Statin Lowering Medications Negatively Affect The Patients Recovery With Back Pain?

Human research has also linked statin use to muscle injury which includes back pain. Most physicians now agree that statins can indeed cause muscle pain and weakness in some people. That is in part because many physicians have themselves experienced these symptoms after taking statins.

The side effects most commonly associated with statin use involve muscle cramping, soreness, fatigue, weakness, and, in rare cases, rapid muscle breakdown that can lead to death. Often, these side effects can become apparent during or after strenuous bouts of exercise. Although the mechanisms by which statins affect muscle performance are not entirely understood, recent research has identified some common causative factors. As musculoskeletal and exercise specialists, physical therapists have a unique opportunity to identify adverse effects related to statin use.

When there are such symptoms as aches, fatigue, and pain that are symmetrical, affect the large muscles, and occur within two weeks after the start of treatment and disappear within two weeks after withdrawing it, the likelihood that the patient is experiencing a statin-related adverse effect is very high.

What Does Research Show In Regards To How Statins Cause Back Pain?

People taking cholesterol-lowering drugs called statins are 30 percent more likely to develop a severe back disorder. The back disorders include bulging discs and narrowing of the spinal column; both of which can cause severe pain, numbness or loss of function. Statins have a long list of potential side effects. This is a new and surprising addition.

Also, the analysts found that people who used a statin for at least four months were 27 percent more likely than non-users to be diagnosed with a back disorder during this time. Such disorders include spinal problems such as spondylosis and intervertebral disc disorders. Researchers suggest that statin use might contribute to the muscle pain often associated with these back problems.

Older studies have shown that up to six out of ten patients taking statins experience side effects; these may include cataracts, liver damage, erectile dysfunction, fatigue, mental confusion and muscle pain. There is great debate among doctors over whether the benefits of statins are worth the severe numerous side effects, or whether high cholesterol is even associated with cardiovascular disease.

What Does Research Show In Regards To How Statins Negatively Affects Cardiac Muscle?

When you have too much LDL cholesterol in your body, it can build up in your arteries, clogging them and making them less flexible. Hardening of the arteries is called atherosclerosis. Blood doesn't flow as well through stiff arteries, so your heart has to work harder to push blood through them. As plaque builds up in your arteries, over time, you can develop heart disease.

Plaque buildup in coronary arteries can disrupt the flow of oxygen-rich blood to your heart muscle. This may cause chest pain called angina. Angina isn't a heart attack, but it can warn that you're at risk for a heart attack. A piece of plaque can eventually break off and form a clot, which can block blood flow to your heart, leading to a heart attack, or to your brain, leading to a stroke.

If you have muscle pain while you take a statin, tell your doctor right away. Your doctor may take you off of the statin for a while to see how your body responds. Although your muscle pain could be caused by the drug, it might be caused by something else.

There are also things that you can do to help reduce your pain. For example, avoid exercising too much. This aggravates muscle aches. Also, avoid using over-the-counter pain relievers. These drugs usually aren't effective at relieving muscle pain from statins.

What Does Research Show In Regards To How Statins Negatively Affect Skeletal Muscle?

Muscle pain and weakness is actually the most common side effect of statin drugs and is thought to occur because statins activate the gene atrogin-1 gene, which plays a key role in muscle atrophy. In severe cases, a life-threatening condition called rhabdomyolysis, in which your muscle cells break down can also develop.

However, muscle pain and weakness are often downplayed as a minor side effect of statin drugs, and one that typically goes away within a couple of weeks of stopping the drugs. In reality, as this new study points out, if you're experiencing any muscle pain when taking statin drugs, it could be because the structural damage is occurring, and this damage may occur even when tests for a protein thought to signal injury are normal.

Further, the damage may persist even after statin use is halted, meaning these drugs may cause permanent muscle damage.

Folks, this is in no way a minor side effect or nuisance. Muscle pain and weakness may be an indication that your body tissues are actually breaking down -- a condition that can cause kidney damage.

One thing is for sure. You should not ignore symptoms of pain and muscle weakness if you are taking statin drugs, as they can deteriorate into even more dangerous conditions, including death.

Finally, Keep track of any new symptoms that develop when you begin taking a statin and report them to your doctor. Some symptoms may go away as you continue to take the medication. If you're taking the statin preventively, your doctor may try to determine if your symptoms are actually due to the statin by suggesting a brief holiday from the drug to see if they disappear when you're not taking it. However, don't stop taking a statin without telling your doctor. Although there are no proven remedies for statin-related muscle pain, exercise may help.

There is some evidence that people who have exercised regularly before taking statins are less likely to experience muscle pain and cramping. Although, gentle stretching may relieve muscle cramps, beginning a new vigorous exercise regimen while taking a statin may increase the risk of muscle pain.

CHAPTER 11: INFLAMMATORY SYNDROME - HOW TO COUNTERACT THE EFFECTS OF THIS SILENT KILLER

BATTLING A NEW EPIDEMIC

Now that you are familiar with some of the common factors that wreak havoc on your system, let's now mention what exactly enters your system when influenced or prone to it.

The term "inflammation", is basically an immune reaction triggered by our systems to prevent any infection by bacteria or damage e.g from injuries. If we examine human history itself, we will find out several bacterial infections and disorders that spread to whole populations but people were able to vanish them. Some of these past disorders include, smallpox, influenza, typhoid fever, and bubonic plague, which are almost extinct today.

While the majority of the above bacterial illnesses have almost vanished, nowadays, we have to face a whole new epidemic. There are multiple health issues today that shave off your quality of lives and well-being like such as, breathing problems, memory issues/alzheimer's, allergies, autoimmune disorders, skin problems, and many more. All these issues that especially affect the Western population aren't caused by bacteria like in the past but from inflammation.

In the past two decades, the frequency of degenerative diseases has been constantly on the rise. Researchers have found that inflammatory disorders have been affecting Americans at an alarming rate because of poor diet habits and induced levels of stress and anxiety. The level of inflammation is at its peak has almost grown to an epidemic. Without any substantial changes to our diet and lifestyle patterns, the country will keep on suffering from diseases like cancer, heart problems, diabetes, Alzheimer's and the list goes on.

WHAT ARE THE EFFECTS OF INFLAMMATION ON THE SYSTEM

When we use the word "inflammation", we usually think of symptoms like "heat", "high temperature", "Irritation", "swelling" and pain somewhere. When a lesion gets inflamed, we can see with our own eyes the inflammation. However, inflammation is not always externally visible like that. The physical signs of "secret" inflammation do emerge but at a much later stage, sometimes when it's too late.

Chronic (long-term) inflammation leads multiple issues in our systems. All sorts of inflammatory disorders may pop up and become a population in our bodies. A person who goes through chronic inflammation, becomes exposed to further health deterioration from diseases and even aging acceleration.

DISORDERS TRIGGERED BY INFLAMMATION

There are various health issues connected with inflammation. Some of the most commonly emerging ones are numerous kinds of arthritis. Arthritis is a broad term that refers to various kinds inflammations in the joint area. Some of the most frequent/common kinds of inflammation-triggered arthritis are:

- Rheumatoid arthritis
- Polymyalgia Rheumatica
- Bursitis
- Shoulder Tendinitis
- Gouty Arthritis

Other stressing body problems targeting the bones and joints of our body, that haven't been yet confirmed to be caused by inflammation but they are still under investigation are:

- Osteoarthritis
- Fibromyalgia
- Neck and back pain (in the muscles)

Shockingly enough, the World Health Organization reveals that over 13 millions of people annually lose their lives from cardiovascular disorders. The cancer rates are also alarmingly big, with 8 millions of people losing their lives from cancer annually. Both of these dangerous disorders are caused by chronic inflammation. So in order to control the likelihood of developing such disorders, we must adopt some healthier diet and lifestyle changes.

Heart disorders separately were to blame for 25% of the deaths in the U.S last year and numbers of people affected are constantly on the rise.

Almost 50% of the deaths linked to heart disorders were a result of chronic inflammation. The numbers may seem exorbitant and unbelievable but they are shockingly true. Inflammation is a huge factor contributing to heart problems.

Based on *National Institute of Health* findings, inflammation is a very vital factor for the development of heart disease and its aggravation. The same goes for other serious and chronic health disorders like cancer and diabetes.

FOODS THAT LEAD TO INFLAMMATION

For those affected by inflammation, diets rich in carbs and low in protein intake can be destructive. As a matter of fact, we've witnessed multiple times that such high carb and low protein diets lead to inflammation while the opposite diet (low carbs/high protein intake), actually keeps inflammation under control and all the negative side effects connected to it.

Every individual organism differs from the other, and thus it is important to spot all the signs and symptoms we experience when we take certain foods. We will offer you a diet against inflammation with all the proper foods to eat later in this report, but at this point, let's delve in a few details.

Processed sugars and foods with an elevated Glycemic Index (G.I), in reality raise insulin levels and trigger an immune system response. There is a communication between inflammatory mediators (prostaglandins, cytokines), and insulin or blood sugar amounts. Studies reveal that when specific stressors emerge, insulin triggers an inflammatory reaction within the system.

Some of the worst foods that trigger an inflammatory response in the body are:

No 1: Sugar/Sweets. High amounts of sugar consumption have been associated with overweight issues, inflammation, and chronic inflammatory diseases like Diabetes Melitus.

No 2: Typical vegetable oils for cooking and baking. Oils with a high omega-6 fatty acid/low omega-3 acid ratio, also lead to inflammation.

No 3: Trans fats. These fats are typically found on junk food/fast food meals. They are also associated with inflammation, resistance to insulin, and other chronic disorders.

No 4: Non-organic milk and dairy products. Non-organic dairy products can also result in inflammation, especially in the female population, due to the hormones and allergen ingredients they contain.

No 5: Red or processed meat. Eating red and processed meat e.g corned beef cans, is also associated with immune reactions that lead to chronic inflammation within our systems. There is also a clean connection between processed meat consumption and cancer risk, backed-up by many scientific trials.

Other types of foods suspect of causing inflammation are grains/flour, alcohol, synthetic food preservatives, and grain-fed meats. All the above foods should be avoided inf nay signs of inflammation emerge.

LINK BETWEEN STRESS AND INFLAMMATION

Going through chronic emotional, mental, and physical stress affects inflammation in the system to a very high degree. In reality, when the system is exposed stress, cortisol levels start to rise within the body.

Cortisol is specifically a steroid hormone that is produced in response to high levels of stress. This may occur from real stressful events or an unhealthy diet or lifestyle. Concerning inflammation, the stress reaction that starts to develop to relieve the body from tolerating such circumstances isn't switched off. Chronic stress is tied to chronic inflammation responses.

In fact, chronic stress has a negative impact on various body functions. For example, it raises blood pressure and hypertension eventually. Chronic blood pressure also puts blood vessels under a tremendous amount of stress. Strokes and heart failures are a common phenomenon in people suffering from chronic inflammation because of inflammatory responses triggered non-stop.

Stress can really "eat" you! Thus, it is vital to learn ways to deal with high stress levels so that you avoid chronic inflammation. Some valuable relaxation methods include:

- Mild exercise
- Yoga/Meditation
- Consuming healthy and nutrient-dense foods
- Learning ways to keep emotional tranquility
- Breathing exercises

INFLAMMATION TREATMENT OPTIONS-THE HARSH ADMINISTRATION OF ANTI-INFLAMMATORY PILLS

The protocol of treatment in response to inflammation is the prescription of anti-inflammatory medicine. The most typically administered drugs in this case are those that provide relief from pain (pain-relievers).

Not long ago, the *American Geriatrics Society* has taken off nearly all non-steroidal and anti-inflammatory drugs from their guide of suggested drugs for people 75+ who experience chronic pain. It was found out that these drugs are overly prescribed, more than necessary and this may lead to negative side effects on the health of older people. Researchers have found that commonly used pain-relievers like ibuprofen, naproxen, and aspirin are not really beneficial for those going through chronic pain. Due to the research conducted on older subjects, researchers are also seeking to examine the excessive administration of NSAIDS in younger subjects as well.

Anti-inflammatory drugs are aimed to lessen pain and discomfort, minimize swelling, and control inflammation symptoms. They are speculated to help with the development of inflammatory disorder, but they don't always function as intended. Anti-inflammatory substances for pain relief feature NSAIDS such as Ibuprofen and Aspirin. Other substances are the ones called corticosteroids (cortisone, prednisone), and numbing pain relievers.

Typically, anti-inflammatory drug substances demonstrate exaggerated side effects. For instance, the consumption of cortisone for extended periods of time can lead to serious problems with bone strength and integrity. Those experiencing asthma symptoms should also seek an alternative treatment option due to negative side effects from anti-inflammatory drugs. Many chronic takers of NSAIDS also develop stomach ulcers and internal bleeding because of the mucus development blocking attributes of these pharmaceuticals. The gastric wall is further exposed to stomach acid in those who consume NSAIDS for longer periods of time to fight inflammation.

Alternative medicine methods approach the matter of inflammation from another perspective. Instead of prescribing synthetic drugs to hinder inflammatory reactions, they suggest the use of vitamins/nutrients and lifestyle changes. While it's true that some vitamins and nutrients have powerful antioxidant and anti-inflammatory properties, they may not completely eradicate the problem. Alternative medicine adopts a more natural way to treatment of the issue as opposed to taking artificial drugs, but doesn't often consider the trigger cause of inflammation.

Further evaluation needs to be performed to find out the exact leading cause of inflammation. It's not holistic or beneficial to only treat the symptoms, but it's just as important to pinpoint the leading culprit of inflammation.

NSAIDS AND THEIR IMPACT ON INFLAMMATION

NSAIDS (Non Steroidal Anti Inflammatory Drugs) are often prescribed against inflammation. These may differ in power and lasting effects on the system. Prostaglandins are a family of chemical substances released by system cells that trigger inflammation in the system when required.

The enzyme responsible for making these Prostaglandins goes by the name "COX" or (Cyclooxygenase). It is also further divided into 2 enzymes: COX-1 and COX-2. Both of these enzymes trigger the release of prostaglandins which lead to inflammation as a result. NSAIDS actually work to block the activity of such enzymes and control the effects of prostaglandins within the system. This eventually leads to long-term inflammation control. However, prostaglandins that guard the stomach lining and enhance blood clotting are also decreased, which results in stomach ulcers and internal bleeding in the region.

NSAIDS when taken excessively, can interfere with physiological COX-1 activity. NSAIDS also hinder the cyclooxygenase pathways. COX-1 is typically produced by normal functioning. The COX-1 stays stabilized under physiological circumstances. In case an NSAID like Aspirin enters the system, COX-1 becomes acetylated and its arachidonic acid pathway is hindered. The process of acetylation is the culprit behind aspirin's anti-clotting and blood-thinning action.

One of the most frequently used NSAIDS is aspirin, which also prevents blood clotting and eventually inhibits strokes and heart failures in people with a heightened risk of experiencing these conditions. NSAIDS though interfere with the physiological activity of heart, kidneys, and stomach due to their action.

INFLAMMATION TESTING-BLOOD EXAMINATION

In those who suffer from long-term inflammation, there is an existing protein secreted by the inflammation region that travels through the bloodstream. One of the common blood tests to find out inflammation is CRP (C-reactive protein test). This test can pinpoint any heightened levels of the protein, which is considered a sign of inflammation.

In several situations when an individual suffers from chronic inflammation which leads to a serious disorder like cancer, arthritis, diabetes, heart failure, or connective tissue (muscle, joints, bones, ligaments) disease, the CRP levels are elevated. These levels are precisely detected through blood testing.

Homocysteine amounts in the blood can also be determined from blood testing. Homocysteine is an acid that is produced by the system physiologically when we consume excessive amounts of red meat. When homocysteine levels are abnormally elevated, the person is a high risk of developing heart problems, atherosclerosis, heart failure, stroke and even Alzheimer's disease.

WHAT'S THE KEY CULPRIT OF INFLAMMATION?

Researchers and medical experts keep on examining the leading cause of inflammation. With so many contributing factors and issues linked to our diets, it's no surprise that gut inflammation has a vital role to play here. We will explain the matter in more details in a later section, but at this point, we should be aware that there is a clear connection between the gut and inflammation. We will examine beyond the natural ways of treating its effects, but study the leading causes behind such symptoms.

Based on scientific evidence, Leaky Gut Syndrome may be the leading cause of many digestive tract diseases like IBS, Crohn's Syndrome, and celiac disease. It can also be the culprit behind the onset of various inflammatory disorders like asthma, allergies, arthritis, and chronic heart problems and disorders.

Practical/holistic medicine takes into consideration the triggering causes of a disorder and doesn't just provide a remedy for the treatment of the symptoms. It is vital to examine all these triggering causes that result in gut and digestive diseases. Gut diseases and syndromes may originate from food sensitivities, leaky gut, and other immunity factors, as stated formerly. We will examine the leading causes in more detail, in a later section.

By addressing inflammation, from a more practical perspective, unlike allopathic or alternative treatment options, we can determine the triggering cause of this modern epidemic. We better know the truth before it's too late!

CHAPTER 12: THE DESTRUCTIVE EFFECTS OF SUGAR

What happens when we take substances that are not prescribed by our doctors yet we consume them without actually realizing it? Sadly, the average American consumes 2-3 pounds of sugar on a weekly basis. The number may seem exaggerated at first, but if we take into account that many types of sugars are sneakily "hidden" in multiple types of foods, such a high amount is not surprising at all. Processed sugar is often found in the form of white sugar (sucrose), corn syrup, and dextrose. These processed and concentrated kinds of sugar are often found in breakfast cereals, bread, jams, butters, condiments/sauces, peanut butter, pies, tomato sauce, and a broad range of processed and pre-made meals.

The average sugar intake in the U.S separately, has risen from the formerly 25 pounds/per individual annual figure, to almost 135 pounds of sugar intake per person annually. Back in the 19th century, the average sugar intake per person was just 5 pounds annually. The levels of sugar intake kept on rising at alarming rates with no indications of reversal. Another noteworthy realization is that up until the early 20th century, cancer and heart problem rates were totally absent.

The blatant association has been backed-up by late scientific evidence that demonstrates that the more sugar someone takes, the higher the risk of developing health problems later in their lives. From elevated cholesterol levels to lower immunity activity, sugar has a detrimental impact on our system.

Let's examine now all the sugar ingredients and the addictive attributed linked with it and its damaging impact to our systems.

THE G.I (GLYCEMIC INDEX)

In order to acknowledge the mechanism of sugar within our system, we should be aware of the Glycemic Index (G.I) first. Every type of food that contains natural or synthetic sugar or linked to a card, is measured according to its G.I. This G.I index is used as a measure on a scale from 0 to 100 (the highest) in association with the impact of this sugar levels on blood glucose levels. Foods that are ranked with a low G.I are deemed to be more healthy and valuable for our bodies, while those with a high G.I score on the contrary, are considered to be unhealthy and damaging to our system.

When someone takes foods with a low G.I (or low in sugar), they can get some health benefits out of their consumption. Here are just some of the health benefits we can reap from taking low G.I foods:

- Decreased levels of cholesterol
- Controlled risk of developing Diabetes or even total elimination
- Increased energy levels
- Controlled cravings and hunger episodes
- Raises sensitivity to insulin
- More stable body weight and loss of excess fat

- Lower risk of developing heart diseases

For the purpose of guarding your system against the detrimental effects of sugar in your system, it's essential to be aware of the G.I score of various foods you are taking. Foods with a low G.I score release controlled amounts of sugar at more gradual speed in your system compared to foods with a high G.I score. The gradual release of sugar in the blood, helps keep energy levels stabilized and prevents those infamous sudden sugar spikes which lead to energy crashes throughout the day. You will realize this happens to you and others, when you take high amounts of sugar after lunch time. If you took a high in sugar food during noon hours, you will most likely feel sleepy and ready to take a nap by 2 a.m.

The blood sugar levels raise to their peak in around on hour after you eat a high sugary food, drink or high carb meal and then they fall suddenly after that hour passes. This is the culprit of energy crashes and tiredness after one hour or so of consuming something high in sugar. The "sugar crash" as we know it, is actually pretty common.

LINK BETWEEN SUGAR AND CHOLESTEROL

Based on the findings of a University of Vermont study, there is connection between high blood lipid levels and sugar intake. The study further demonstrated that heightened consumption of sugar was also associated with elevated triglyceride levels and decreased levels of HDL (the beneficial) cholesterol. The research outcomes were so evident that the American Heart Association has also validated these findings in public.

The study performed demonstrated people taking raised amounts of sugar or high amounts of processed white sugar (sucrose). When these people took excess amounts of sugar, their triglyceride levels were heightened whereas their good HDL levels were quite low within their blood. Very low HDL levels are associated with a heightened risk of developing heart disease.

At this point, why HDL cholesterol is beneficial for the system and why sugar has a destructive effect on our systems? You may already be aware that not all cholesterol/fat lipids are actually bad for your system. This notion is actually true, but having no sufficient amounts of good HDL cholesterol can be very destructive to your heart and system. HDL is actually the beneficial cholesterol that circulates through the blood and carries mini lipoproteins that that act synergistically to cleanse the blood stream.

HDL performs the following beneficial functions in the system:

- HDL cleanses and strips from the bad lipids/LDL cholesterol through circulating small assistant lipo-proteins.
- HDL recycles bad cholesterol by sending it to the liver to be handed and reformed.
- HDL acts a maintenance group that repairs the internal linings of the blood vessels that became destructed through a procedure known as "atherosclerosis". HDL is the most ideal factor for cleansing the blood from bad cholesterol and keep the body functioning at its peak capacity. It actually unblocks the internal linings of blood vessels and prevents destruction coming from toughening of arterial walls (atherosclerosis), as stated earlier. Individuals who take high-sugary foods and drinks, smoke, are inactive, or experience obesity problems, are more prone to develop heart disorders that those following healthier lifestyle habits. Overall, people with high levels of

good HDL cholesterol are much less likely to develop heart problems whereas those with low HDL scores in their blood are more prone to develop heart disorders, among other health issues.

SUGAR AND ITS DETRIMENTAL IMPACT ON THE IMMUNE SYSTEM

A study performed during the 1970s, demonstrated that a persons own white blood cells required amounts of Vitamin C to process and expel out of their system bacteria, viruses, and other intruders. White blood cells need 50X the amount of Vitamin C, to go through this phase within a cellular level. For the purpose of finding out how fast this procedure happens (also known as phagocytosis), a phagocytic index may be utilized. In the 70s, scientist Linus Pauling demonstrated through his trials that blood cells require adequate amounts of Vitamin C. He has found out that when someone has caught a cold, high amounts of Vitamin C are needed to treat cold/make it heal faster. Due to the fact that both Vitamin C and sugar have similar chemical forms, they antagonize each other when blood sugar levels get raised in the bloodstream. They two in reality rival each other to penetrate the cell. Therefore, when there are higher amounts of sugar present in the bloodstream, due to sugar intake, this will allow fewer amounts of Vitamin C to penetrate the cell. When we take high amounts of sugar, the immune system function will come to a sticky end.

Up to this point, we have explained the common cold and how a rise in blood sugar levels hinders Vitamin C from penetrating the cell walls to fight the common cold virus but what happens in other disorders? The same principle is also applicable. Insulin struggles for its way to penetrate the cell when higher amounts of it are already existing within the cell than Vitamin C. This principle also applies to inflammatory disorders like diabetes, cancer, heart problems, and asthma. The common denominator here is the high intake of sugar.

Common sugars have been demonstrated to worsen health problems such as:

- Cancer
- Cardiovascular problems
- Arthritis
- Osteoporosis
- Diabetes
- Development of gallstones

LINK BETWEEN CANCER AND SUGAR

Regulating the provision of sugar in the bloodstream is very valuable for tackling cancer. There has been this old yet widespread notion that "cancer feeds on sugar". This has been proven to be accurate, but we need to understand better the mechanisms of such association.

In the early 1930s, German Scientist Otto Warburg, was awarded the Nobel prize for being the first to discover the fluctuating energy metabolism of cancer cells as opposed to that of healthy cells. The final finding emerging from his trials was that cancer cells use sugar at a much more elevated pace than normal healthy cells. The more sugar exists in the system, the more it is taken by the cells of the body. So in other words, the sugar actually is a source of food for cancer cells and can contribute to their spread and development at a later stage.

As emerging from the above study, cancer treatment protocols nowadays are aiming to control blood sugar levels in numerous ways.

Physicians often suggest a healthy low-sugar diet, physical activity and drug administration in individuals suffering from cancer.

SUGAR AND ITS CONNECTION WITH MENTAL HEALTH

Besides sugar bearing an impact on various physical functions of our system, it also affects mental health. Numerous trials examining sugar and its connection to the worsening of mental health disorders have been conducted by Malcolm Peet, an established and renowned mental health/psychiatry researcher. Dr. Peet found a definite connection between high sugar intake and mental health disorder through extensive trials and studies on patients suffering from schizophrenia. Based on the outcomes of his studies, there is a clear association between elevated glucose levels and high risk of developing mental health problems like depression and schizophrenia.

Sugar has a detrimental effect on the central nervous system and mental health as a result. It actually downgrades mental activity by hindering the function of an important growth hormone called "BDNF", which leads to various chemical responses in the system that ultimately trigger long-term inflammation. The inflammation process hinders the activity of the immune system and leads to mental/brain issues. Concerning the growth hormone BDNF, when amounts of this hormone fall to below physiological ranges, there is a higher risk of developing depression or schizophrenia.

Through extended and in-depth studies, Dr. Peet discovered that long-term inflammation in the system is triggered by high intake of sugar, which suppresses the normal activity of the immune system and makes it lose its power to fight back. Additional evidence from studies also validates the connection between high sugar consumption and aggravation of mental health disorders.

There are several studies featured in the British Journal Of Psychiatry that demonstrate a connection between diets high in sugar and mental health issues like stress, anxiety, depression, and others. These trials didn't concentrate on issues triggered by inflammation, but demonstrated instead that people who take high amounts of sugar on a regular basis, are more likely to develop anxiety, depression, and possibly other mental health disorders. Additionally, sugar leads to a fast spike in adrenaline levels which triggers episodes of induced stress, anxiety, hyperactivity, and struggle to maintain focus. Scientists have revealed that following a diet that's nutrient-dense and low in sugar balanced mood levels and our ability to concentrate. People who took wholesome foods as a part of their diet regimes, were shown to experience better mood and deal with stressful situations more efficiently.

THE IMPACT OF SUGAR ON OUR KIDS

Sugar sadly is making its effects shown in the health of children, by being a contributing factor, based on various study findings, that's tied to high rates of child obesity and other health problems arising from high sugar intake. Child health experts across the world, are worried that excessive sugar intake in kid diets is damaging to their health. While sugar alone isn't destructive, it's high consumption leads to an increased gain of body fat and raises the risk of childhood obesity.

Based on Baylor University of Texas studies and trials, the heightened tendency of childhood obesity rates over the past years is clearly associated with a high intake of sugar by kids over the same timeframe. We can't neglect the reality that our kids take excessive amounts of sugar and eventually become obese and fat. The majority of sugar intake originates from candy, breakfast cereals, sweetened granola bars, processed juices, and fizzy drinks.

The childhood obesity rates are constantly rising up remarkably every year and our children suffer from poor health. Pediatricians sadly reveal that now, more than ever, children are treated for health problems that used to bother adults mostly in the past. Children visit a doctor's office for symptoms connected with elevated blood pressure, heart problems, and diabetes. All these conditions are associated with a high sugar intake.

SUGAR ADDICTIVE ATTRIBUTES IN RELATION TO THE BRAIN

Some folks have very strong cravings and urges to consumer sweets or at least foods high in sugar and carbs. Researchers of the Monell Chemical Senses Center of Philadelphia, support that people were brought to this world with a varying appetite for sugar. During trials carried out in fetuses in the wombs of their mothers, sweet compounds were passing through the amniotic liquid. This lead to the fetus taking higher amounts of amniotic fluid than those indicated. There were measured carried out to address excessive levels of amniotic fluid in the womb. The measures were able to address the issue, but also showed that infants may later develop a higher preference for sweets.

When there is a high sugar intake, some changes emerge in the brain. Animal trials demonstrated alterations in the dopamine levels of the brain, emerge after the intake of sugar. Like in the case of drug addiction, animals that were provided with intermittent sugar intake have demonstrated a remarkable rise of levels of dopamine in the brain.

While people who frequently take sugar, do not experience the tremor and chills or harsh withdrawals drug addicts experience when they withdraw the use of drugs, people do experience strong cravings for sugar. There is no special study, up to this point carried out to examine better sugar's addictive characteristics but there is one evident point: sugar cravings emerge which in turn lead to excessive consumption of sugar, which ultimately contributes to the development of body fat and obesity, heart issues, and even death in extreme stages.

BE CAUTIOUS OF CONCEALED SUGARS

Studies conducted by University of Vermont's nutrition department, found out that only a small minority of Americans actually comply with the standard guideline of taking no more than 150 calories from sugar daily. This guideline has been published by the AHA (American Heart Association), and functions as a target for individuals to meet by decreasing their sugar intake daily. The small amount of people who are aware of this AHA guideline show a decreased risk for developing heart disorders as opposed to those that exceed the indicated levels of sugar intake per day.

Sugar is sneakily hidden in so many kinds of foods that we have no other option than to read the list of ingredients in every food label to find out any amounts of sugar/sugar forms. Many food labels though are misleading or ambiguous and thus we should be aware of hidden sugars prior buying and consuming a food or taking the food label as it, without closer speculation. There are two general rules when it comes to deciphering food labels:

No 1: Find out any words ending in -ose e.g sucralose, fructose, dextrose,e tc.

No 2: Pay close attention to names like "evaporated cane sugar" or "evaporated cane juice".

Additionally, in many food labels and especially on canned fruits, veggies and even savory foods like meats or condiments, there is the word "syrup" in the ingredients list or words ending with -ose e.g sucralose, dextrose, or fructose. Any of these should be avoided. Furthermore, high fructose corn syrup is a sugar form you better totally stay away from. These sugars found in common foods are artificial and processed sugars which may lead to various health problems when taken excessively.

But the main source of hidden sugar in someone's diet isn't sweets, but soft drinks/sodas. These include, colas, soda pops, juice cocktails, and other drinks with a high sugar content. Processed foods are also the second leading cause of elevated sugar in our bodies. Following a healthier and cleaner diet can help us get rid of excess sugar in our systems. Drinking plain water or tea in the place of fizzy drinks and eating natural wholesome foods instead of processed junk make a great start for cleansing our diet and bodies.

CHAPTER 13: EAT YOUR WAY OUT OF PAIN THE ANTI-INFLAMMATION DIET

Much of the pain and inflammation an individual suffers is biochemically conditioned.

It makes sense. The pain medication provides relief by affecting biochemistry. Is there a way to naturally influence the chemistry of the body to reduce pain and inflammation? The answer is yes! There are foods that increase inflammation and there are foods that can reduce inflammation. Understanding this will allow you to make lifestyle changes that reduce or even eliminate the number of painkillers you should take.

What is inflammation?

Inflammation is the body's response to an injury. When the tissue is injured, there are a number of chemical changes that occur; we call these changes inflammation. An injured and inflamed body area undergoes a continuous change as the body heals and repairs itself.

When an injury occurs, the body responds with the four features of inflammation: pain, heat, redness, and swelling. Think of a bee sting.

First, there is the bite, the initial wound. The body's response to the injury causes redness, heat, and swelling, as well as mild additional pain. The blood vessels in the area of the lesion expand and the white blood cells produce chemicals such as prostaglandins, cytokines, interleukins, and leukotrienes, which cause these inflammatory changes; This happens within 30 minutes of the injury. The white blood cells then migrate to the area. If the injury is not too severe, the blood vessels will return to normal within six to eight hours and repair can begin.

What causes inflammation?

Inflammation occurs due to certain chemicals produced by white blood cells in response to an injury. Sometimes there is an exaggerated response to the injury and the inflammation can produce pain that is not proportional to the injury. Medications can inhibit inflammation by disrupting the production of inflammatory chemicals, but they also slow down the healing process. However, they can naturally reduce the inflammation without slowing the healing process.

You may have heard the names of some chemicals involved in inflammation drug advertising. Three examples of these pro-inflammatory chemicals are prostaglandins, cytokines, interleukins, and leukotrienes. Medications that treat allergies and relieve pain and inflammation affect these chemicals. Similarly, diet and supplements can also affect the amount of these chemicals and the inflammation that they produce.

Chemistry of inflammation

The chemistry of pain has been extensively studied. Much of the research involves measuring the number of chemicals involved in the inflammation. Scientists can determine if food can cause inflammation or reduce inflammation by measuring the chemicals produced by inflammation. For example, mice were examined at the University of Buffalo. Mice have been genetically bred to age quickly, have immune system abnormalities, and are prone to developing autoimmune diseases. In a diet containing omega-3 fatty acids and vitamin E, the mice produced lower levels of vitamin C inflammatory cytokines compared to mice that did not receive omega-3 and omega-3 fatty acids.

Other research has shown that sugar, refined foods, and processed foods can increase the chemicals that cause inflammation. Insensitivity to insulin can lead to inflammation. Insulin insensitivity is the result of too many refined carbohydrates (refined sugars and starch products like sweets, pasta, and white bread). Insulin-insensitive people tend to be overweight and usually carry excess weight in the abdomen, thighs, and buttocks. Studies have shown that overweight people tend to produce more inflammatory chemicals than people who are not overweight.

The fact is the lifestyle you live and the food you eat can affect how much pain you feel. The research appears in the Journal of the American Medical Association

(2004; 292: 1440-1446) shows that the Mediterranean diet can protect the lining of blood vessels and reduce inflammation. In the study, the chemicals that produce inflammation were actually reduced with the diet.

Most diseases are the result of inflammation. Heart disease, Crohn's disease, allergies and even cancer are inflammatory diseases.

Controlling the inflammation not only reduces pain but also improves overall health.

A physiotherapist from the Danish Olympic Committee recently conducted a study to document the anti-inflammatory properties of diet and supplementation. This was tested in 1996 for the first time in a group of rowers of the Danish Rowing Association. The study found that a combination of antioxidants and essential fatty acids can be an effective treatment for inflammation in wounds commonly known as "tennis elbow" and "Gulf elbow".

Antioxidants neutralize free radicals. This limits their destructive effects, so athletes should ensure that they receive sufficient levels of antioxidants to protect themselves from stress injuries. Essential fatty acids are important because they promote the production of Type 1 and Type 3 prostaglandins in the body (chemicals that neutralize pain and inflammation).

The amount of antioxidants in your diet is especially important if you want to reduce pain and inflammation. Another aspect of your diet that can reduce pain and inflammation is the type of fats and oils that you consume.

According to a study by Dr. Med. Richard Sperling of Brigham and Women's Hospital can reduce fish oil's inflammatory substances produced by white blood cells. If you have an inflammatory condition such as rheumatoid arthritis (RA), the type of fat in your diet can alter the immune system's inflammatory response.

The intake of polyunsaturated omega-3 fatty acids (PUFA type fish oil) in many industrialized countries is relatively low. Research has shown that increasing the amount of omega-3 fatty acids in the diet different health problems, including atherosclerosis, cardiac arrhythmias, multiple sclerosis, major depression, autoimmune diseases and inflammatory diseases In general, it has been shown that omega-3 PUFAs cause pain in patients with rheumatoid arthritis, inflammatory bowel disease, and other painful conditions.

Anti-inflammatory diet

Much of the pain and inflammation an individual suffers is biochemically conditioned. It makes sense. The pain medication provides relief by affecting biochemistry. It is logical to think that other ways of influencing the body's biochemistry (such as diet and nutritional supplements) can also affect pain and inflammation. There are foods that increase inflammation and there are foods that can reduce inflammation. Understanding this will allow you to make lifestyle changes that reduce or even eliminate the number of painkillers you should take.

We can use our knowledge about the chemistry of inflammation and develop a diet that really relieves pain and inflammation.

Drink a lot of water every day:

You need water to keep your cells hydrated and protected, to prevent waste, and to ensure the health of your mucous membranes. The most important thing when drinking water when it comes to pain is the fact that water attracts the cartilage and needs enough water for your joints to function properly. Dehydration causes excessive joint wear and may result in disc injury. Drink more water and less soft drinks, coffee, tea or juice.

Eat a lot of vegetables:

Many mean that at least one percent of the food (volume) you eat. Vegetables are very high in fiber, vitamin C, folic acid, antioxidants, and minerals. Some practitioners believe that we do not live on the food we eat; we live on energy in the food that we eat. They believe that raw food is better than cooked food. We will not tell you to avoid hot food, but it is a good idea to increase the amount of fresh and raw foods in your diet. They offer many health benefits such as:

Vegetables are very rich in antioxidants. You may have heard of bioflavonoids or carotenes; these are pigments that give fruit and vegetable color. They are also antioxidants that protect the cells of the solar plant. When consumed, they also provide their cells with antioxidant protection.

A fiber in vegetables reduces the absorption of fats and toxins. Eating enough fiber can help you lose weight and normalize cholesterol and blood pressure.

Vegetables nourish the normal flora, which in turn nourishes the lining of the gastrointestinal tract, produces vitamins and inhibits yeast and other unwanted organisms.

Vegetables accelerate intestinal transit time, reducing gut toxicity and preventing irritation of the gastrointestinal lining.

Vegetables contain folic acid, which is needed to produce serotonin (to prevent depression and overeating), increase energy and reduce the risk of heart attack.

The minerals in vegetables help to prevent osteoporosis. Minerals are also important enzymatic cofactors, so most of the important functions of the body depend on minerals.

Eating vegetables can reduce the incidence of cancer and heart disease, increase energy and mental clarity, reduce the problems caused by intestinal and liver toxicity, and reduce the symptoms of allergies, asthma, arthritis, skin problems, digestive problems, chronic sinusitis pain, and many other health problems,

Ideally, 80% of the volume of food you eat should be vegetables. Corn and potatoes are not considered vegetables. The fruit is good for you as well; it is a good source of vitamin C and fiber. Eating vegetables is striking here because when people are supposed to eat more fruits and vegetables, they tend to increase their consumption of fruits, not the consumption of vegetables.

To get well, it is recommended to eat 80% of fresh products (and nuts and raw seeds) and 20% of other foods. Eating four vegetables and two fruits in a food rich in starch and protein meal (proportional to volume) approaches this number. Yes, the instance has 3 ounces of protein per day; you need 12 ounces of vegetables and 8 ounces of fruit per day. You can also get 3 ounces of cereal, but you should not eat it with meat.

The reason why this report works well here is that most Americans tend to eat a lot of grain and protein and not many vegetables. We also tend to combine starch and proteins. Changing these eating habits often has dramatic health effects.

Maintaining health is easier. If you do not have major health problems, you should eat 60% fresh fruits and vegetables, nuts and seeds to maintain your health. This results in one protein, one starch, two vegetables and one fruit. If you have 6 ounces of protein then you need 12 ounces of vegetables and 6 ounces of fruit per day. You may also eat 6 ounces of grain, but you should not eat it with meat. When you eat like this, fruits and vegetables dominate your diet; if they are fresh and raw, much better. If you can get organic products, it will eliminate the stress that pesticides have on your body.

Avoid fried foods, Trans fats, partially hydrogenated oil and hydrogenated oil.

Over time, we find more and worse things about hydrogenated oil and fried foods. Hydrogenation is the way the food industry transforms liquid oils into solid fats. (Trans fat). Although hydrogenated oils are responsible for a variety of health issues, the food industry uses them because they give packaged foods a longer shelf life than if they were made with natural oils. Hydrogenation produces Trans fats that have been linked to a range of health issues, including:

The pain and inflammation worsen in patients who consume hydrogenated oils. They chemically prevent the formation of natural anti-inflammatory substances that the body normally produces. If you have chronic pain or recent injury, be sure to avoid hardened oils. In addition, muscle fatigue and skin problems are also associated with hydrogenated oils.

Most chronic diseases are due to inflammation. Because Trans fats increase inflammation, they are also associated with a variety of health problems. Women with a higher Trans fatty acid content in their cells develop breast cancer much more often than women with a low Trans fatty acid content. High Trans fats are associated with coronary heart disease. Lately, much has been written that links inflammation to heart disease. Trans fats are incorporated into cells and make them less resistant to chemicals, bacteria, and viruses. This could be a source of immune system problems. There may be a link between Trans fatty acids and ADD, depression and fatigue. The brain and nerve tissue are fatty. Some researchers believe that trans fatty acids when incorporated into nerve cells affect function and cause problems such as ADD and depression.

Most chips and fried snacks contain hydrogenated oils. Hydrogenated oils are contained in a large amount of packaged foods such as biscuits, cereals, and even bread. They are often found in margarine (margarine is far worse for you than butter); Mayonnaise; and many bottles of salad dressings. Read the labels

All fats are not bad for you.

Permissible fats are raw (not roasted) nuts, extra virgin or extra virgin olive oil and avocados.

Avoid refined sugar:

The average American eats 150 pounds of refined sugar a year. Compare that to 17 pounds a year consumed in England in 1750. Refined sugar increases the production of insulin and adrenal hormones and can cause the following health problems. First, sugar increases inflammation. Sugar increases insulin production and insulin can also increase the presence of inflammatory chemicals.

The increased production of adrenal hormones causes the excretion of essential minerals.

Sugar consumption consumes vitamins B and C.

Eating too much sugar aggravates many of the problems associated with emotional stress.

Sugar nourishes the yeast and other single-celled organisms in the intestine that multiply. These organisms produce toxins, irritate the lining of the gastrointestinal tract and replace the normal and beneficial flora, thereby eliminating the benefits of beneficial bacteria.

Eating sugar causes changes in blood sugar levels. The glucose level rises immediately after the consumption of sugar, resulting in insulin production by the body. Excess insulin generates more sugar cravings.

Eating sugar causes insensitivity to insulin. More sugar is consumed; more insulin is produced, etc. This emphasizes the pancreas and sets the stage for adult diabetes.

There is a connection between sugar intake and hypercholesterolemia. Patients with Syndrome X (high cholesterol, high LDL, low HDL and high triglycerides) often have the problem of consuming sugar and refined carbohydrates.

Sugar can cause or worsen allergies, sinusitis, asthma, irritable bowel, candidates, migraines, fatigue, depression and even heart disease.

Avoid refined carbohydrates:

The average American gets 50% of its refined carbohydrate calories. Refined carbohydrates are grains that have eliminated fiber, vitamin E, B vitamins, bran, and germs. In other words, the nutrients have been eliminated and the strength is retained. They all create the same health problems caused by refined sugar. Go back and read the problems caused by refined sugar and discover that the list of refined starches is exactly the same.

Refined carbohydrates fill up, but not with vitamins and minerals. This highlights your digestive system and your endocrine system. Eating refined carbohydrates consumes valuable vitamins and minerals.

People often eat refined carbohydrates because they are low in fat and falsely think that because they are "complex carbohydrates", they are really good for you. Refined carbohydrates are white bread, white rice, and noodles that are not labeled with whole grains. Read the labels on the bread. Wheat bread with a black bread label is usually not a whole grain. If the label says fortified white flour, you will not get wholegrain. Use brown rice instead of white rice.

Avoid chemical additives:

Avoid processed foods and chemicals. The average American consumes 10 pounds of chemical supplements per year. It had devastating effects on our health. The FDA is testing individual additives, but no one has any idea what additive combinations will do for us. Stay away from foods that are packed with chemical additives and you will be much healthier.

Eat slowly, chew your food thoroughly:

Ideally, chew your food until it is liquid. You will be satisfied with less food and you will have better digestion. Their saliva has enzymes that facilitate digestion. It is also easier to digest small particles than large ones. Do not chew your stress on your digestive system and can lead to poor absorption of nutrients, digestive problems such as flatulence and flatulence, and promote the growth of harmful bacteria in the digestive tract.

Never skip meals:

The omission of meals examines your adrenal glands and therefore can aggravate any inflammatory disease. It can also make you feel tired and eventually gain weight.

If you need more energy or if you have a chronic health problem, you should follow this diet. Although there is a lot of controversy about the alkaline ash content (even for advocates who disagree with the details), patients do well if they follow it. There are some controversial concepts that are added to the basic diet, such as the combination of food and alkaline ashes, but try it. This diet seems to help many health problems.

Summary of anti-inflammatory diet:

Drink a lot of water every day.

Fresh vegetables should dominate your diet.
Avoid fried foods, partially hydrogenated oil and hydrogenated oil.
Avoid refined sugar.
Avoid refined carbohydrates.
Avoid chemical additives.
Eat slowly and chew the food well.
Never skip meals.

If you have a chronic health problem or pain, 80% of your diet should be fresh (fruits, vegetables, nuts, and seeds) and 20% may be other foods (animal products, protein, whole grains). In practical terms, eat four vegetables and two fruits of a starchy food and protein (proportional, by volume).

If you are in good health, save it by consuming 60% fresh produce and 40% other foods (protein, animal products, whole grains, etc.). Specifically, this means one protein, one starch, two vegetables and one fruit (proportional to volume).

If you can, follow some additional rules. Eat mainly raw products. It's good to eat cooked food, but we follow Dr. Reams that we do not live on the food we eat, we live on energy in the food we eat. It is better to eat raw foods than to eat cooked foods. Alcohol and caffeine should be limited.

Do not eat proteins and carbohydrates together. Do not eat fruit with cereals or other foods. It's an old concept called "alkaline ash diet," which is controversial and has written many strange things about it. It turns out that adhering to these two simple rules, along with the rest of nutritional advice, is especially helpful for people with digestive problems.

If you follow the basic diet, you can always follow the eating habits. You can eat meat and potatoes, a sandwich with egg whites and whole grains. The extra discipline of "combining food" is often very helpful for people who are trying to lose weight and have many digestive problems or other health problems. You do not have to limit the amount of food you eat, you just have to change the way you think about food. You really need to think about food by fueling your body and not with likes and dislikes. You probably need to plan your meals in advance and not just take food in the race. Try it very strictly for 30 days. Most people can do everything for 30 days. It improves your health and energy and helps you to understand the connection between what you eat and how you feel.

On the next page, we have given you an example of a five-day diet. They are just a few suggestions to help you choose what to eat and not a strict diet. Use it as a guide.

Why not take supplements?

You may have noticed that supplements such as antioxidants and omega-3s have been mentioned in this report. There are even herbs like willow bark, curcumin and others that can naturally reduce inflammation. It is a good idea to seek professional advice before taking supplements. If you take a substance that you do not need, it will not help. The need for supplementation varies from person to person. You can call our office and we can help you with an individual program.

Day 1	BREAKFAST	Apple with almond butter
	LUNCH	Tuna (mix it with olive oil, chopped onion, and celery). Serve it on celery stalks, carrot sticks and/or cucumber slices. You can also include tomato and onion slices
	DINNER	Sweet potato (you can use a small amount of clarified butter-- or slice it and cook it in a casserole with sliced apples in pineapple juice), large green salad (oil and vinegar dressing), mixed cooked vegetables.
	SNACKS	Any fruit, nuts or any vegetable
Day 2	BREAKFAST	Oatmeal
	LUNCH	Turkey, large green salad
	DINNER	Brown rice, cooked vegetables, large green salad
	SNACK	Any fruit, nuts or any vegetable
Day 3	BREAKFAST	Quinoa
	LUNCH	Chicken vegetable soup, large green salad
	DINNER	Chicken, large green salad, cooked vegetables
	SNACK	Any fruit, nuts or any vegetable
Day 4	BREAKFAST	Melon

	LUNCH	Hummus, tabouli, goat feta cheese, and cucumber slices
	DINNER	Beef vegetable soup, large green salad
	SNACK	Any fruit, nuts or any vegetable.
Day 5	BREAKFAST	Vegetable omelet (chopped onion, spinach, tomatoes and bell peppers [if nightshades are not a problem for you]).
	LUNCH	Stir-fried vegetables and brown rice
	DINNER	Broiled salmon, avocado, and a green salad
	SNACK	Any fruit, nuts or any vegetable.

CHAPTER 14: A NUTRITIONAL APPROACH TO REDUCING SPINAL INFLAMMATION

Hyaluronic Acid:

Hyaluronic acid (HA) is a naturally produced non-sulfated glycosaminoglycan (GAG) non-protein substance with repeating -1,4-D-glucuronic acid and -1,3-N-acetylglucosamine units with different physicochemical characteristics. HA possesses high viscoelasticity, moisture retention capacity, biocompatibility, and hygroscopic characteristics.

HA chains can offer high viscosity at concentrations as low as 0.1 percent. HA works as a lubricant, shock absorber, joint structure stabilizer, and water balance- and flow resistance regulator due to these characteristics.

The fluids of the eyes and joints contain hyaluronic acid. It works as a lubricant and a cushion in the joints and other tissues. Various types of hyaluronic acid are utilized for various reasons. Hyaluronic acid may also impact how the body responds to damage and contribute in the reduction of edema. Its key role is to retain water in order to keep your tissues lubricated and moisturized.

Knee osteoarthritis can be treated with high molecular weight (HMW) hyaluronic acid (HA). Hyaluronic acid injections are FDA-approved in the United States for a variety of conditions, including osteoarthritis. Hyaluronic acid is also frequently taken orally and applied to the skin for wound healing and a variety of other diseases.

HA is a component of ECM that promotes cell proliferation, motility, and morphogenesis. HA is found within cells and has been linked to cellular functions. Type B synoviocytes are the primary producers of HA molecules within the joint cavity. HA (a disaccharide polymer) may have a length of 25,000 disaccharide repetitions and a MW of 5,000–20,000,000 Da.

Benefits Of Hyaluronic Acid Benefit For Your Knee Degeneration:

Hyaluronic acid is used by doctors to treat arthritis-related joint pain. Hyaluronic acid is also present in synovial fluid in the joints, where it keeps the gap between your bones lubricated.

The bones are less prone to grind against each other and induce pain when the joints are lubricated. The hyaluronic acid in synovial fluid degrades over time, contributing to joint soreness and rigidity.

People suffering with osteoarthritis, a kind of degenerative joint condition caused by wear and tear on the joints over time, can benefit greatly from hyaluronic acid supplementation.

Osteoarthritis (OA) is a condition that causes a progressive loss of cartilage over years and decades.

The primary signs of this condition are joint pain and soreness. Although OA may affect any synovial joint, OA of the knee joints is the most common and causes the most discomfort. The articular cartilage undergoes considerable structural, mechanical, and matrix changes with age-related OA, including mild fibrillation of the articular surface and a reduction in proteoglycan monomer size and aggregation.

OA is a disease that affects the entire joint, including the articular cartilage, chondrocytes, synovial capsule and membrane, and periarticular tissues (connective and muscular) (such as ligaments, tendons, and in the menisci).

The MW of HA and mode of administration are also known to influence the degree of anti-inflammatory, immunomodulatory, analgesic, and anti-OA actions of HA.

Hyaluronic acid can be administered intravenously into the joints. Joint pain and stiffness can be reduced by injecting hyaluronic acid into the joint. The US FDA has authorized it as a medical product for this purpose.

Because it minimizes systemic exposure and potential unwanted side effects, intra-arterial (IA) treatment is said to be more effective than oral or IV administration. A number of studies have looked into a treatment with HA, and it has been used as OA therapy in humans for decades. IA injection of HA into OA joints can improve mobility, articular function, and pain by restoring the rheological characteristics of the SF and promoting endogenous production of a higher MW and presumably more functional HA.

In general, hyaluronic acid injections appear to be safe when used according to the directions.

However, some persons may experience unpleasant side effects including allergic responses to hyaluronic acid. People who receive hyaluronic acid injections may have the following adverse effects, which should resolve within a week: soreness, redness, itching, swelling, and bruising. These adverse effects are more likely to be caused by the injection process than by the hyaluronic acid solution itself.

Taking Hyaluronic Acid Orally For Your Knee Degeneration:

Hyaluronic acid is generally safe to take by mouth. Allergic reactions are possible, although they are uncommon. It has been proven that taking 80–200 mg daily for at least two months considerably reduces knee pain in patients with osteoarthritis, particularly those under the age of 40.

Recent research suggests that combining oral hyaluronic acid supplements with injections might greatly enhance pain relief and extend the duration between treatments.

Glucosamine:

Glucosamine is a naturally occurring chemical in cartilage. It is classified as an amino sugar. It acts as a building block for a wide range of functional molecules in your body. It is well known for its involvement in the development and maintenance of cartilage in your joints. Glucosamine may also be present in animal and nonhuman tissues, such as shellfish shells, animal bones, and fungi.

Glucosamine supplements are available in several forms, including glucosamine sulfate, glucosamine hydrochloride, and N-acetyl glucosamine. Glucosamine is extracted from shellfish shells or synthesized in a laboratory.

Some glucosamine supplements include additional substances such as chondroitin sulfate, shark cartilage, or methylsulfonylmethane (MSM).

Benefits Of Glucosamine For Your Knee Degeneration:

The body uses glucosamine to create other compounds that help to develop tendons, ligaments, cartilage, and the fluid that surrounds joints. The fluid and cartilage that surrounds joints provide cushioning. Taking glucosamine may assist to enhance cartilage and fluid surrounding joints and/or prevent joint degeneration.

Oral glucosamine sulfate is used to treat a painful disease caused by cartilage inflammation, degradation, and eventual loss (osteoarthritis).

Glucosamine is used by the body to produce and repair cartilage. Cartilage is a connective tissue that is flexible, strong, and rubbery that covers the bones in the joints. It cushions the bones and keeps them from rubbing together.

As people age, their cartilage becomes less flexible and begins to degrade. This can result in discomfort, inflammation, and tissue destruction, as seen in osteoarthritis. Glucosamine is found naturally in the body, although levels decline as people age. The decline may contribute to joint degeneration over time.

One of its primary functions is to promote the proper growth of articular cartilage, which is a smooth white structure that surrounds the extremities of your bones where they meet to create joints.

Articular cartilage, in conjunction with the lubricating liquid known as synovial fluid, reduces friction and allows bones to slide easily and smoothly across one another. Glucosamine is believed to stimulate the formation of certain chemical molecules, such as collagen, which are critical structural constituents of articular cartilage and synovial fluid.

Taking glucosamine supplements may preserve joint tissue by avoiding cartilage degradation, especially in athletes. One research, for example, found that ingesting 1.5–3 grams of glucosamine daily for three months reduced cartilage degradation in collegiate footballers and professional rugby athletes.

Glucosamine is essential for the formation of glycosaminoglycans and glycoproteins, which are the building blocks of numerous joints, including ligaments, tendons, cartilage, and synovial fluid. It has been found that the manner in which certain elements of your joint are formed and maintained contributes to the development and progression of osteoarthritis. Giving glucosamine can both delay and restore cartilage degradation.

Glucosamine supplements are commonly used to treat a variety of bone and joint disorders. The majority of scientific study on glucosamine has been on one specific type known as glucosamine sulfate.

This chemical has been extensively researched for its potential to treat osteoarthritis (OA), rheumatoid arthritis (RA), and osteoporosis symptoms and disease progression. Taking glucosamine sulfate tablets on a regular basis may provide an effective, long-term management for OA by considerably lowering pain, preserving joint space, and delaying disease development.

When taken orally, glucosamine sulfate is considered safe for most individuals to consume for up to three years. When administered for up to two years, glucosamine hydrochloride may be safe for most individuals. N-acetyl glucosamine may also be safe to take for up to 6 months. The normal glucosamine dosage is 1,500–3,000 mg per day, which can be taken all at once or in lesser quantities throughout the day.

Some minor adverse effects of glucosamine include bloating, nausea, diarrhea, and constipation. Due to a lack of information on its safety, you should avoid using glucosamine if you are pregnant or breastfeeding.

Also, keep in mind that glucosamine may have a little hypoglycemia impact in those with type 2 diabetes, although the risk is minimal. Before using glucosamine, see your doctor if you have diabetes or are on diabetic drugs.

Methylsulfonylmethane (MSM):

Methylsulfonylmethane is a chemical compound found in fresh raw foods such as fruits, vegetables, and meat. MSM is a white crystalline chemical that includes 34% sulphur and is used to treat diseases. MSM is made from dimethyl sulfoxide (DMSO), an organic sulfur compound that is also utilized as a food supplement.

It can also be manufactured in a laboratory to make powdered or capsuled nutritional supplements.

MSM is commonly used in alternative medicine and by those seeking a natural solution to treat knee degeneration pain, reduce inflammation, and enhance immunity.

MSM tablets are commonly used to treat arthritis, joint pain, knee degeneration pain, and muscle recovery after exercise.

Benefits Of Methylsulfonylmethane (MSM) For Your Knee Degeneration:

Many of MSM's advantages are related to its anti-inflammatory properties. Inflammation has a role in a variety of medical disorders, including arthritis, allergies, and skin diseases. MSM may be able to decrease or eliminate various symptoms by lowering inflammation.

One of the most typical uses for MSM is to alleviate knee joint or muscle pain. It has been found to help patients suffering from joint degeneration, which is a prevalent cause of pain in the knees, back, hands, and hips.

Joint degeneration can reduce your quality of life by restricting your movement and mobility. MSM has been found in studies to considerably decrease inflammation in the body. It also prevents cartilage degeneration, which is a flexible substance that covers the extremities of your bones in joints.

According to one study, taking a supplement containing 1,200 mg of MSM for 12 weeks reduced joint pain, stiffness, and inflammation. Another study discovered that taking a glucosamine supplement with MSM markedly reduced lumbar stiffness and soreness when moving, as well as greatly improved quality of life.

MSM supplementation may aid in the relief of post-workout knee discomfort and tissue stress. Some small studies indicate that it may be beneficial in this regard. Exercise's energy needs can produce oxidative stress in muscles and tissues. This may cause acute pain and discomfort following an exercise. By lowering inflammation and oxidative stress, MSM can naturally speed up muscle recovery after intensive exercise.

As an anti-inflammatory substance, MSM can be extremely useful. It suppresses NF-kB, a protein complex in your body that is involved in inflammatory reactions. It also lowers the production of cytokines including tumor necrosis factor alpha (TNF-) and interleukin 6 (IL-6), which are signaling proteins associated with systemic inflammation.

MSM can also boost glutathione levels, a powerful antioxidant generated by the body. As a result, MSM may inhibit the production of inflammatory molecules such as TNF- and IL-6 while increasing levels of the potent antioxidant glutathione. As a result, MSM may be quite effective for knee degeneration pain.

Arthritis is a common inflammatory disorder that causes joint pain, stiffness, and a limited range of motion. Because MSM has potent anti-inflammatory characteristics, it is frequently used as a natural alternative to medicines to alleviate arthritic symptoms. It can boost the efficiency of other common arthritis supplements such glucosamine sulfate, chondroitin sulfate, and boswellic acid.

According to one study, combining MSM with glucosamine and chondroitin was more beneficial than glucosamine and chondroitin alone in reducing pain and stiffness in persons with knee osteoarthritis.

Knee pain can also be caused by a weakened immune system. A weakened immune system exposes your body to infections and illnesses. MSM is essential for the functioning of your immune system.

MSM, for example, may be useful in lowering oxidative stress and inflammation, both of which can decrease immunity. MSM may alleviate immune system stress since it is efficient at lowering levels of inflammatory chemicals such as IL-6 and TNF-. It helps in the production of glutathione, your body's main antioxidant. It may also benefit in increasing quantities of this critical chemical.

Adequate glutathione levels are critical for general health and immune system function. So, by lowering inflammation and raising glutathione levels, MSM may help enhance your immune system.

MSM is considered safe at doses of less than 3,000 milligrams (mg) per kilogram (kg) per day, according to the Food and Drug Administration (FDA). Most individuals may take 3 g per day of capsules, powder, or cream without experiencing major adverse effects, however people should see a doctor before taking the supplement on a long-term basis. MSM supplements are available in pill or powder form.

Taking more MSM than recommended does not appear to improve outcomes. MSM is thought to be safe and well tolerated, with few negative effects. The FDA and other major regulatory organizations have awarded it the Generally Recognized As Safe (GRAS) status.

However, some people who are sensitive to MSM may develop minor problems such as nausea, bloating, and diarrhea. It may produce minor skin or eye irritation when applied to the skin.

L-Arginine:

L-arginine is an amino acid that is required for protein synthesis and is commonly used in circulation. The protein can be used by the body to help develop muscle and repair tissue.

It can be acquired naturally through diet and as a dietary supplement. Plant and animal proteins high in L-arginine include dairy products, beef, chicken, fish, and nuts. L-arginine is one of several amino acids required by the body to work properly.

Nitric oxide is produced in the blood by L-arginine. Nitric oxide works in the circulation to dilate blood vessels, which may assist with some cardiovascular problems.

Under normal conditions, the body manufactures L-arginine naturally. People also acquire more L-arginine from their usual diet. Red meats, fish, dairy, and eggs all have low levels of L-arginine, which helps the body restore its resources.

A person's requirement for L-arginine may occasionally exceed the body's ability to create or absorb it naturally. This is especially true for the old or those suffering from certain medical conditions. In these circumstances, patients may be given synthetic L-arginine in the form of pills, injections, or gels. A higher intake may benefit a variety of different health issues.

When your body is affected due to diseases such as infection, trauma, or knee degeneration, your arginine needs drastically rise due to physiologic demands. Under these conditions, your body is unable to meet your arginine requirements, which must be provided from outside sources.

Arginine deficiency during critical illness or following surgery has major consequences, including reduced immune function and blood flow. Arginine supplements are commonly utilized in the clinical setting to address a range of diseases in order to prevent these potential complications. L-arginine also increases the production of growth hormone, insulin, and other hormones in the body.

Benefits Of L-Arginine For Your Knee Degeneration:

L-arginine can help with knee degeneration pain. In the body, L-arginine is turned into a molecule known as nitric oxide. Nitric oxide causes blood arteries to dilate, which improves blood flow.

L-Arginine reduces bone erosion in RA via inhibiting the RANKL/RANK/Traf6 pathway and altering cellular metabolism during osteoclastogenesis. Immunometabolism Arginine's activity may therefore assist in the reduction of joint inflammation and damage in RA.

In serum-induced arthritis, L-arginine treatment decreases clinical symptoms, bone degradation, and osteoclast counts. Furthermore, L-arginine concentrations in the blood of rheumatoid arthritis (RA) patients have been found to be lower.

L-arginine is a substrate for various enzymes in the cell, including Arg-1. Several studies have shown that Arg-1 has an anti-inflammatory action and can help with inflammatory diseases.

L-anti-inflammatory Arginine's properties promote muscle repair. The ability of l-arginine to inhibit cytokine release by macrophages in muscle, including TNF-, IL-1, and IL-6, implies that this molecule may interfere with inflammatory pathways generated during the dystrophic process.

L-arginine dosage varies greatly depending on the condition being treated. Overall, research has demonstrated that L-arginine is safe and well tolerated when taken as a supplement, even when used regularly for a year or more.

However, when used in high dosages of 9 grams or more per day, it might induce undesirable side effects. Indigestion, nausea, headache, bloating, diarrhea, gout, blood irregularities, allergies, airway inflammation, aggravation of asthma symptoms, impaired insulin sensitivity, and low blood pressure are all possible adverse effects of L-arginine.

Because higher dosages of L-arginine might produce a rise in stomach acid, it may aggravate heartburn, ulcers, or digestive trouble caused by drugs. Furthermore, L-arginine may worsen herpes symptoms in patients. L-arginine may interact with some medicines, including blood pressure pills, diabetic medications, and erectile dysfunction treatments.

References:

1. Alberto. *"Effectiveness And Utility Of Hyaluronic Acid In Osteoarthritis"*. Retrieved from Nih.gov: https://www.ncbi.nlm.nih.gov/pmc/articles/PMC4469223/

2. Steven. *"Recent Advances In Hyaluronic Acid Based Therapy For Osteoarthritis"*. Retrieved from Nih.gov: https://www.ncbi.nlm.nih.gov/pmc/articles/PMC5814393/

3. Jean. *"Role Of Glucosamine In The Treatment For Osteoarthritis"*. Retrieved from Nih.gov: https://www.ncbi.nlm.nih.gov/pmc/articles/PMC3456914/

4. Toru. *"Effects Of Glucosamine In Patients With Osteoarthritis Of The Knee: A Systematic Review And Meta-Analysis"*. Retrieved from Nih.gov: https://www.ncbi.nlm.nih.gov/pmc/articles/PMC6097075/

5. Kim, L. *"Efficacy Of Methylsulfonylmethane (MSM) In Osteoarthritis Pain Of The Knee: A Pilot Clinical Trial"*. Retrieved from Sciencedirect.com: https://www.sciencedirect.com/science/article/pii/S1063458405002852

6. Eytan. *"Efficacy Of Methylsulfonylmethane Supplementation On Osteoarthritis Of The Knee: A Randomized Controlled Study"*. Retrieved from Bmc.com: https://bmccomplementmedtherapies.biomedcentral.com/articles/10.1186/1472-6882-11-50

7. Valerio. *"L-Arginine, Asymmetric Dimethylarginine, And Symmetric Dimethylarginine In Plasma And Synovial Fluid Of Patients With Knee Osteoarthritis"*. Retrieved from Nih.gov: https://www.ncbi.nlm.nih.gov/pmc/articles/PMC3852624/

CHAPTER 15: THE POWER OF THE PRO-ADJUSTER

Developments in computer and engineering technology have indeed been able to incorporate Chiropractic to evaluate and heal the human body in ways that had never been seen before. As a result, the human being's ability to eliminate pain and reach maximum nervous system performance has never been more vital.

Luckily, we possess the technology and procedures to meet the demands imposed on the spine and neurological system. For example, chiropractors can diagnose nervous system abnormalities using the pain-free and efficient Pro-Adjuster by delicately evaluating the spine to see whether specific vertebrae move too smoothly or too firmly.

This article shows how this contemporary Pro-Adjuster technology can help you ease back discomfort and regain your mobility.

Every day, breakthroughs occur in this technological era. Chiropractors specialize in spinal and limb manipulations to aid you in regaining equilibrium in your back. More therapy options become available as the field improves.

The ProAdjuster is a cutting-edge chiropractic tool. It's an advanced chiropractic technique built on NASA's space technology. It's a gadget that goes over your spine's vertebrae. It locates any vertebrae which are out of line using digital technologies. The Pro-Adjuster detects and adjusts spinal subluxations. Subluxation correction gives comfort and resolves these vexing or unpleasant issues.

Chiropractors used to depend on X-rays or contact, physically running their hands along the spine, searching for any anomalies. The ProAdjuster, on the other hand, detects any anomalies and gently touches the vertebrae to push them into perfect alignment.

The Pro-Adjuster correctly assesses if the vertebrae are out of place by exerting very low mechanical stress on the spine. This power is about the same as pressing your fingers on a tabletop. In addition, the vibration transmitted to the Pro-Adjuster enables the computer to analyze the location of each vertebra in detail, providing the Doctor with significantly more knowledge regarding your spinal condition than was previously accessible. Consequently, you will receive a more excellent standard of care than was initially offered.

Engineer Dr. Joseph Evans' company Sense Technology invented the ProAdjuster system. The ProAdjuster is a chiropractic instrument that provides moderate, successful, and effective treatment without the twisting and rapid motions that some patients detest about hand adjustments.

Before the muscle can react normally, a gentle force is delivered into the vertebra to verify motion. Then, it is directed back to the piezoelectric sensor, which detects the reflecting point and sends it to the computer for analysis. Isn't it amazing? This is the same technique and device that NASA scientists often used to test the condition of the ceramic cooling tiles on the exterior of the space shuttle during the space agency.

NASA originally developed the Pro-Adjuster technology to be used on spacecraft to see if the rivets on spaceships could resist the shocks of take-off and landing. The aviation sector has utilized this technique and structural engineers to assess metal wear in aircraft and bridge structures. In addition, this space-age equipment is being adopted in the practice of chiropractors to identify and correct spinal manipulations successfully.

Chiropractors may now leverage this cutting-edge technology to assess the proper operation of the human body.

Contrary to common assumption, treatment is frequently simple and appears entirely ordinary and un-dramatic. The Doctor can decide how to cure your condition based on various criteria, including the patient's medical history and x-rays.

Chiropractic involves a thorough assessment of the body's joints to see whether and where there is a functional misalignment. A chiropractor can physically return the joint to its ideal position and flexion if the dislocation is found and identified. To stabilize the issue, it may need one or several treatments.

A chiropractor uses pressure to correct misplaced vertebrae and enhance nervous system function throughout a spinal adjustment. Previously, changes were made by hand, but new technology has made it possible to automate the process in recent times. In addition, the technique has become more exact thanks to computer-assisted equipment. The ProAdjuster is one such sophisticated tool.

The ProAdjuster includes computer software that reads data and a hand-held gadget that analyses joint motion and performs the correction.

A ProAdjuster treatment is soothing and more pleasant for so many of our patients than a standard adjustment. In addition, patients stay sitting throughout the therapy, and because the instrument only applies the pressure that each specific joint requires, the treatments are often softer and more accurate.

The Pro-Adjuster pleasantly prods the body into alignment and facilitates healthy spinal activity by combining conventional chiropractic expertise with advanced technology. It identifies and treats abnormalities in the neurological system, which regulates all physiological functions. Inflammation may cause the organ to malfunction whenever the neurological system is unbalanced. As a result, chronic discomfort, disease, and a decline in health might happen if nothing is done to address the imbalance.

The Pro-Adjuster diagnoses nervous system issues by gently evaluating the spine to see whether specific vertebrae are moving too smoothly or firmly. The nerve function might be compromised if the spine is overly stiff. A chiropractor checks for joint stiffness when personally evaluating your spine, but the Pro-assessments Adjusters are much more exact than manual treatments.

For starters, you won't be hearing any cracking noises coming from your spine. Instead, the Pro-Adjuster uses gentle oscillating vibration to gradually correct the misaligned portion of your spine, relieving nerve "pinching." Consequently, pain, tension, migraines, digestive issues, and other symptoms are alleviated. For your comfort, the pressure level may be carefully regulated and modified. When the imbalance is fixed, the Pro-Adjuster detects it and immediately stops the treatment at the precise moment. That's why the procedure is painless, quick, and efficient.

The ProAdjuster360 properly measures and analyzes joint motion using cutting-edge automated therapy technology, then offers pleasant, precise adjustments depending on every patient's information. Following therapy, the post-treatment study confirms better joint mobility alterations. In addition, the utilization of data throughout each visit provides total trust in the treatment and administration of the patient's individualized treatment regimen for both the patient and therapist.

The current version of the ProAdjuster 360 system can analyze and cure joints other than the spine, such as the shoulders, elbows, wrists, hands, hips, knees, feet, and ankles. The ProAdjuster360's ergonomic, automated, and reliable technology delivers a pre-treatment assessment, accompanied by specially directed adjustments and a verified post-treatment study that culminates in a measurable change in joint conformity.

Dr. Chapman (a chiropractor) has collected a list of research that back up the treatments he offers in his practice. We've included them here to understand what the study says about the ProAdjuster and the advantages of the standard treatment alternative.

Simple Pelvic Traction Gives Inconsistent Relief to Herniated Lumbar Disc Sufferers

"Serial MRI of 20 patients treated with the decompression table shows in our study up to 90% reduction of sub ligamentous nucleus herniation in 10 of 14. Some rehydration occurs detected by T2 and proton density signal increase. However, torn annulus repair is seen in all."

Eyerman, Edward MD. Simple pelvic traction gives herniated lumbar disc sufferers inconsistent relief. Journal of Neuroimaging. Paper presented to the American Society of Neuroimaging, Orlando, Florida 2-26-98.

Decompression, Reduction, and Stabilization of the Lumbar Spine: A Cost-Effective Treatment for Lumbosacral Pain

"Eighty-six percent of ruptured intervertebral disc (RID) patients achieved 'good' (50

89% improvement) to 'excellent' (90-100% improvement) results with decompression. Sciatica and back pain were relieved." "Of the facet arthrosis patients, 75% obtained 'good' to 'excellent' results with decompression."

C. Norman Shealy, MD, PhD, and Vera Borgmeyer, RN, MA.Decompression, Reduction, and Stabilization of the Lumbar Spine: A Cost-Effective Treatment for Lumbosacral Pain. American Journal of Pain Management Vol. 7 No. 2 April 1997

Surgical Alternatives: Spinal Decompression

"Results showed that 86% of the 219 patients who completed the therapy reported immediate resolution of symptoms, while 84% remained pain-free 90 days post-treatment. In addition, physical examination findings showed improvement in 92% of the 219 patients, and remained intact in 89% of these patients 90 days after treatment."

Gionis, Thomas MD; Groteke, Eric DC. Surgical Alternatives: Spinal Decompression. Orthopedic Technology Review. 2003; 6 (5).

A Clinical Trial on Non-Surgical Spinal Decompression Using Vertebral Axial Distraction Delivered by a Computerized Traction Device

"All but two of the patients in the study improved at least 30% or more in the first three weeks."Utilizing the outcome measures, this form of decompression reduces symptoms and improves activities of daily living."

Bruce Gundersen, DC, FACO; Michael Henrie, MS II, Josh Christensen, DC. A Clinical Trial on Non-Surgical Spinal Decompression Using Vertebral Axial Distraction Delivered by a Computerized Traction Device. The Academy of Chiropractic Orthopedists, Quarterly Journal of ACO, June 2004

Disc Distraction Shows Evidence Of Regenerative Potential In Degenerated Intervertebral Discs As Evaluated By Protein Expression, Magnetic Resonance Imaging, And Messenger Ribonucleic Acid Expression Analysis

"Distraction results in disc rehydration stimulated extracellular matrix gene expression, and increased numbers of protein-expressing cells."

Guehring T, Omlor GW, Lorenz H, Engelleiter K, Richter W, Carstens C, Kroeber M. Department of Orthopaedic Surgery, University of Heidelberg, Germany. Disc distraction shows regenerative potential in degenerated intervertebral discs as evaluated by protein expression, magnetic resonance imaging, and messenger ribonucleic acid expression analysis. Spine. 2006 Jul 1;31(15):1658-65

What Conditions Can The Pro-Adjuster Treat?

The Pro-Adjuster uses technology to relieve stress from adversely impacted nerves, making it ideal for persistent back discomfort. The Pro-Adjuster relieves pain and tension throughout the body and headaches, digestive issues, and more. The therapy is mild, regulated, constant, and quantifiable, and it can be used to treat:

- Car Accident Injuries
- Lower Back Pain
- Headaches / Migraines
- Pinched Nerves
- Numbness in Arms / Hands
- Neck Pain
- Arm / Leg Pain
- Fibromyalgia
- Carpal Tunnel Syndrome
- Muscle Spasms

Are There Any Contraindications To Getting Treated With The Pro-Adjuster?

Chiropractic contraindications are exceedingly uncommon, and chiropractic treatment is incredibly successful (and inexpensive!) in treating various spinal pain disorders, notably back pain, neck pain, sciatica, migraines, and whiplash. Yet, there are times when caution calls for a diversion.

If you have any of the following, don't go to a chiropractor: osteoporosis, Arm or leg numbness, stiffness, or weakness. Your spine is cancerous. If your problems do not improve, even slightly, after four weeks of starting therapy, you may be sent to a different type of clinician for more diagnostic tests, treatment, or co-treatment.

Note that what might be beneficial can also be harmful in health care. Your chiropractor is taught to check for chiropractic contraindications and cause no damage. Every medical procedure has some risk, yet Chiropractic is among the safest medical treatments available.

How Many Sessions Are Needed To See Benefits From The Pro-Adjuster?

An individual seeking ProAdjuster treatment for the goals of preventive or wellness should expect a 9 to 10-week treatment regimen. The routine is one session each week, comprising 20-40 minutes.

Your chiropractor will research each of your sessions, modify you with the Pro-Adjuster, and then revaluate. The alterations in your spine will be seen right away. In addition, your issue regions will be displayed on the computer screen, along with the impacted organs in the body. This provides you with a comprehensive grasp of your issue. In addition, it will inform you how your treatment is progressing and the extent to which your disease has been resolved.

The Doctor will next use the device to re-evaluate the spine, with a post-analysis presented on display. You'll be able to correlate the before and after measurements and see how much has changed. Since each appointment is founded on a new assessment of your spine, each therapy will improve on the one before it!

Final Words

Medications aren't always enough. They may provide immediate comfort, but they will fade off, and you don't want to become dependent on prescription medicines. Chiropractic adjustments can help you. You should anticipate even positive benefits with the ProAdjuster. The Pro-Adjuster machine identifies the optimal correction mode for your situation before applying a regulated force to the imbalance. The therapy is reliable and safe for people of all ages.

WE hope you found our Pro-adjuster guide helpful. Do you have any further questions? Let us know in the comments below.

CHAPTER 16: UNDERSTANDING THE BASICS OF DECOMPRESSION THERAPY

Decompression therapy is a non surgical manipulation of the spine, in order to relieve pain and improve spinal function. This procedure would involve stretching the spine with the use of a traction table or any other motorised device that may be similar to it (Gay, 2013). The procedure is non surgical and is usually carried out by a Chiropractor, a trained and licensed medical expert, who specialises in mechanical manipulation of the bone and joints without prescribing drugs or performing surgery.

This decompression therapy is a ground-breaking treatment that involves the careful and mechanical stretching of the spine which is a gentle and non surgical approach to providing instant relief to disc-related pressure which causes the pain, stimulate blood and oxygen flow through the spine which enables the lubrication of the discs hence providing long term healing and improvement of pain symptoms in patients that have suffered from chronic lumbar pains.

Spinal decompression is performed on a traction table with the aid of advanced computer technology. It operates under the same basic principles that chiropractors have been using over the years to stretch the spine and provide effective relief from painful symptoms. This therapy works by slowly and steadily stretching the spinal column to remove the abnormal pressure that had been exerted on the discs that sit between the vertebrae. This stretching action in turn creates a negative pressure inside the discs in the spine that causes them to retract. The process of retraction creates a reverse vacuum that helps to draw protruding disc material back into place. This promotes increased flow of blood into spinal discs encouraging nutrient rich fluids and oxygen to flow inside the spaces which in turn promotes cell renewal, tissue repair and provides for long term healing of lumbar (lower back) pains (Choi et al., 2015).

Spinal decompression, as a procedure, can be carried out both surgically and non-surgically. The surgical procedures are largely classified into two broad types, laminectomy and microdisectomy, both are invasive techniques that can be considered as treatment options if the non surgical procedures fail to achieve the aim and meet the needs of the patients (Wheeler, 2021).

WHO DISCOVERED DECOMPRESSION THERAPY?

Allan Dyer, in 1985 discovered decompression therapy and six years after, he developed VAX-D, the first decompression table. So technically, decompression therapy has been around for over thirty years. The original VAX-D decompression table was controlled by a pneumatic system that gradually applied and released with traction, force that was being applied to the back or legs to reduce muscle spasm (Daniel, 2007). This revolutionary computer-aided technology that aids relief the patient of chronic back pain is FDA-approved. The treatment process is safe and usually lasts for a period of thirty to forty minutes per treatment session. A typical spinal decompression treatment protocol consists of about 12-20 sessions over four to six weeks. However, some conditions may require lesser or more visits depending on the severity of the condition.

THE SCIENCE BEHIND DECOMPRESSION THERAPY

The main theory behind decompression therapy is the traction it provides to compressed structures in the spine leading to relieve of both pressure and pain in the affected regions (Wegner et al., 2013). In spinal decompression therapy, both traction and decompression techniques are applied with the aim of relieving pain and promoting an optimal and enabling environment for conditions such as herniated discs, bulging discs or degenerating discs (Gay, 2013).

A herniated disc refers to a condition that occurs when inflammatory proteins from the disc's inner core leak out. This inflammatory proteins go ahead to cause pain, swelling and discomfort in the back. These inflammatory materials may in turn pinch, inflame or irritate a nearby nerve causing nerve root pains that manifest as sharp and shooting pains, radiating to various parts of the body (Haines, 2018). Typically, a herniated and degenerative disc disease occurs in the cervical spine (neck) and the lumbar spine (lower back region), but it seems to be the most common in the lower back where most of the body movement that involves weight bearing occurs. However, this condition is uncommon in the mid-back region which is the thoracic spine (Haines, 2018).

So basically, since herniated discs slip out of place and cause a depression of the nerves around the area thus leading to chronic pains, what spinal decompression seeks to achieve is to create traction in the spine, which in turn creates space(s) between the vertebras that relieves the pressure on the surrounding nerves. Medications only mask pain symptoms for a short period of time without actually providing a cure or treatment for the condition.

THE STUDIES THAT PROVE THAT DECOMPRESSION THERAPY IS SUITABLE FOR HERNIATED DISCS

According to the Lumberton Chiropractic Health Centre, Texas, there have been more than ten successful research studies that have been carried out on spinal decompression as an alternative procedure to surgery, for patients suffering from herniated, bulging, degenerating and slipped discs that manifests as lumbar pain in the lower back region.

Daniel, in 2007, performed a single controlled randomized trial, comparing the efficacy of spinal decompression using the VX-D machine to the TENS (Transcutaneous Electrical Nerve Stimulation) in the treatment of lumbar (lower back) pains in patients with herniated discs (Daniel, 2007). The herniations of the discs were confirmed using CT (computed tomography) and MRI (magnetic resonance imaging) scans. The treatments consisted of 30-minute sessions, five times per week for four weeks, followed by weekly sessions for four weeks. The control group received TENS for 30 minutes every day for twenty days, followed by weekly treatment for four weeks (Daniel, 2007).

At the conclusion of the study, thirteen out of the nineteen treatment group with VAX-D showed improvement while zero out of the twenty-one control group with TENS showed improvement. At the sixth month follow-up, all nineteen of the original subjects in the treatment group with VAX-D showed remarkable and sustained improvement in lumbar pains while the control group had none (Daniel, 2007).

Another study was carried out by Choi et al., using general traction therapy as the control. Thirty subjects with chronic back pain and intervertebral disc herniation were used, 15 had the spinal decompression therapy (recall that this technique combines both traction and decompression of herniated discs) while the other 15 had the general traction therapy using the lumbar traction device. Both groups received conservation physical therapy three times per week for four weeks. A Visual Analog Scale (VAS) was used to measure the degree of pain in the patients while the Oswestry Disability Index (ODI) was used to measure the degree of functional disability in the patient. The conclusion derived from the study was that spinal decompression therapy and general traction therapy both give significant relief to the patient and are both effective in the management and improvement of lumbar pains associated with intervertebral disc herniation.

However, spinal decompression therapy yielded a larger a larger degree of pain reduction and a higher increase in range of motion compared to the general traction therapy which was the control group. We can therefore attribute this difference in therapeutic outcome to the fact that spinal decompression therapy combines two methods, traction and decompression of the discs while the general traction which was the control applied only one method- the general traction (Choi et al., 2015, Lee et al., 2012, Kang, 2011, Yang, and Ramos and Martin, 1994).

This study conducted by Choi et al., goes ahead to point out why decompression therapy has recorded much success over the years in alleviating lumbar pains with little or no side effects attached to the procedure. One of the reasons while the decompression technique yielded that difference would be because in the act of decompressing the herniated discs there is a realignment of the vertebra that make up the spine in that region (usually the lumbar region), this realignment allows fluids and oxygen to slip their way back into discs between the vertebra allowing for smooth lubrication in the affection area. This method, coupled with the traction which stretches and relaxes the spine, intermittently in a controlled manner thus creating a negative interdiscal pressure in the spine, accounts for its widespread success. Patients who have been living with chronic back pain when introduced to decompression therapy testified of the immediate relief that accompanied the therapy sessions without altering their general work and life routines as the surgery would have (Gay, 2013).

SHORT TERM AND LONG TERM BENEFITS OF DECOMPRESSION THERAPY

Spinal decompression therapy has been a last resort over the years for patients who have tried to alleviate and bring relief to pains in their lower back regions. This group of people must have previously sought relief from medications only to discover that it only brings temporary relief and nothing permanent. The first all-round benefit of this decompression therapy is the non-invasive approach the technique offers. It eliminates the inconvenience associated with its surgical alternative and does not cause a change in lifestyle, habit and work activities as the surgical procedure would. For patients that have been managing their back pains using NSAIDs (Non Steroidal Anti-Inflammatory Drugs) and Opioid analgesics, the adverse effects associated with the long term use of this pain medication which include; liver and kidney impairment(for drugs highly metabolised and excreted by these organs), tolerance and addiction (especially with the Opioid analgesics) would be ruled out with decompression therapy as they would no longer need those drugs to manage the lumbar pains or cervical pains.

The short term benefits of this procedure include;

- Spinal decompression therapy helps to relieve the pressure that pushes the discs in the spine out of place which makes the disc to press and irritate surrounding nerves. The irritation and bulging of surrounding nerves causes the chronic pains.
- Spinal decompression therapy causes remarkably fast relief to chronic back pains. It's amazing how patients would walk in for a therapy session that lasts for almost 30 or 40 minutes and walk out the next second with a significant relief of lower back pains.
- Spinal decompression helps to retract herniated discs. This can bring about both short term and long term benefits in the sense that while the herniated discs would be retracted by a realignment of the spine causing fluids and oxygen to flow back into their original position, lubricating the discs and causing a relief of pain in the short term, consistent and frequent sessions of decompression therapy would lead to a permanent eradication of pain and inflammation in the affected regions.
- Spinal decompression helps to gently stretch the spine, making the discs that had gone out of place to return to the correct position. Stretching of the spine is also relaxing especially because the pain on the lower back is because of the weight bearing capacity of that spinal region (lumbar vertebrae).

The long term benefits would include all the short term benefits taking place consistently over an extended period of time. This can only happen if the patient adheres strictly to his therapy sessions and appointments. On a whole, the most important long term benefit of spinal decompression therapy would be that it has a short recovery time so it enables the patient to still go about his routine activities unlike the surgical alternative that would restrict the patient's movement for a period of time or the medication approach that only mask pain without providing a permanent solution or treatment to the underlying lower back pain.

Also, the patient would not have to spend the rest of their life taking drugs for the chronic pain as it is seen with some chronic diseases such as diabetes and hypertension when the option of decompression therapy is readily available and relatively cheaper, considering the therapeutic, humanistic and economic outcomes of the patient (Yang, 2008).

Overtime, decompression therapy helps the discs in the spine to remain in place instead of migrating outside the intended spots continually (Wheeler, 2021).

WHAT TO EXPECT WITH DECOMPRESSION THERAPY

People who have been living with persistent neck, back or sciatic nerve pain caused by herniated or degenerative spinal discs don't have to live a life dependent on medication or resort to surgery as spinal decompression therapy has shown to give remarkable sustained pain improvement benefits.

Spinal decompression therapy is an effortless but gradual process that is carried out on a motorized table with the upper half fixed while the lower half of the table moves when it is activated by a highly specialized computer. Therefore to treat a disc problem that affects the lower back, a harness is fitted comfortably around the hips while the other end is attached to the lower end of the table near the feet. After the computerized table has been activated, it slides back and forth gently thus lengthening the spine and alleviating the pressure that has been built up in them (Gay, 2013).

Decompression therapy is an advanced chiropractic care that can be trusted with a single decompression session lasting for about thirty minutes. The average decompression treatment protocol consists of an average of twelve to twenty sessions lasting over a period of four to six weeks. After the first therapy session, a significant pain relief would be experienced but it is important that patients follow through with the complete duration of therapy session to ensure sustained and long lasting relief of symptomatic pain in the spine.

However, patients that may have had severe trauma owing to lower back pains, while decompression therapy may be painless for some, it may not be painless for others in his class. The process of stretching and traction of the spine in the region where pain is experienced may cause even more pain and discomfort in the first few therapy sessions. Since a complete treatment protocol consists about twenty or more sessions depending on individual needs of the patients, before a treatment procedure is concluded the patient experiencing traumatic pain must have witnessed some relief as the treatment progressed. It is very important for patient that experienced pain in their first few therapy sessions to be encouraged to follow through their treatment outline to the latter as the pain would significantly reduce as eventually stop before the entire treatment s concluded.

CONTRAINDICATIONS OF DECOMPRESSION THERAPY

Despite the beautiful benefits (both short term and long term) of decompression therapy, they are however some group of individuals who due to their physiological, pathological state or existing deficiencies would not be advised to undergo the procedure of spinal decompression therapy.

They include;

- Pregnant women due to their physical state would not be advised to try decompression therapy. Back pains and Sciatica are common conditions that present during pregnancy and a patient may be tempted to consider decompression therapy in order to relieve the pain. Chiropractic treatment and massages if carried out with care can be advised but because of the traction involved in spinal decompression therapy, a pregnant patient is strongly advised against it. However if the lower back pains persist after the delivery, the consulting physician would recommend a suitable time when the decompression therapy sessions should be commenced.
- Patients with already broken vertebrae should not try decompression therapy. Since decompression therapy involves stretching of the spine in order to realign them, a broken vertebra would only suffer more pain and problems while being stretched and these may partially or totally damage the spine of the patient.
- Patient who because of one reason or the other had to undergo spinal fusion would not be advised to undergo decompression therapy. The manipulation of the spine during the process of decompression may not be suitable for this patient because of the state of their spine. Their physician is however in the best

position to advise them on what other alternatives to try in order to relieve their back pains.
- Patients with existing spinal implants or artificial disc in the spine would not be advised to undergo decompression therapy. Decompression therapy sessions would stretch their implants and artificial discs and push them out of their original positions hence the contraindication.
- Patient with a history of back surgery or patient who have had multiple back surgeries without recovery or significant improvement of pain symptoms would also not be advised to consider the option of decompression therapy. This is because the spine has already been manipulated severally hence the process of spinal decompression therapy would not be suitable as it involves general traction of the spine.
- Patients with significant spinal osteoporosis should not be advised to undergo spinal decompression therapy either in the lumbar or cervical region. This is because there is an increased risk of vertebral compression fractures from the decreased bone density and undergoing spinal decompression may add to that risk. Patients with severe osteoporosis may sustain fractures simply by getting up from a chair or moving from one place to another, or even just sneezing, much more undergoing spinal decompression therapy.
- In general, conditions in which the spine had previously been manipulated or undergone surgery or implantation would cause contraindications for the patients. It is important to look out for these physical states either pre-existing or not before proceeding with decompression therapy as an option for alleviating back pains. The process of decompression therapy involves traction and decompression of herniated discs, their

mechanisms by which they exert their effect is the reason these conditions have to be looked out for before proceeding to treatment.

Decompression therapy as we had earlier stated has recorded widespread successes over the years and has been in use for more than three decades. It has been an effective alternative for patients who did not want to undergo surgery and also for patients who have tried to manage their pains with pain medications without any significant success. Decompression therapy has through the process of general traction of the spine and decompression of herniated discs present also in the spine brought relief to patient suffering from lower back pain by not only providing symptomatic relief but eliminating the root cause of the pain which is the herniated discs that slip out of place, pressing the surrounding nerves thereby causing the pain and the inflammatory proteins that leak out of the discs causing the inflammation and pain. The process of decompression cause the discs to go back into place causing a flow of fluids and oxygen to the discs which serve as lubricating agents for the discs in the spine. The traction of the spine also reliefs the pressure exerted on the nerves in the spine bringing about a permanent solution to the patient.

The understanding of the pathophysiology of disc herniation and pain in the spine especially in the lumbar region helps to understand the mechanism of action of decompression therapy and why it has recorded so much success over the years.

REFERENCES

1. Colin Haines, MD: What's Herniated Disc, Pinched Nerve, Bulging Disc...? 2018 [Spine health]

2. DM, Daniel: Non-surgical Spinal Decompression therapy: does the scientific literature support efficacy claims made in advertising media? Chiropract osteopath.2007;15:7 [Biomed Central]

3. Inge Wegner, Indah S Widyahening and Cochrane Back and Neck group: Traction for low-back pain with or without Sciatica. Cochrane database Syst. Rev.2013 Aug;2013(8): CD003010

4. Jioun Choi, MS, PT, Sangyong Lee, PhD, PT and Gak Hwangbo PhD, PT: Influences Of Spinal Decompression Therapy and General Traction on the Pain, Disability and straight leg raising of patients With Intervertebral Disc Herniation. J Phys Ther Sci.2015 Feb;27(2):481-483

5. Kang DY: The effects of Spinal Decompression Therapy and manual therapy on the pain, flexibility and muscle activity in patients with herniated intervertebral lumbar disc. Korea University, Dissertation of master's degree, 2011.

6. Lee Y, Lee CR, Cho M: Effect of decompression therapy combined with joint mobilization on patients with lumbar herniated nucleus pulposus. J Phys Ther Sci,2012,24:829-832 [Google Scholar]

7. Ralph Gay, MD: Potential Candidates for Spinal Decompression Therapy. 2013 [Spine Health]

8. Ramos G, Martin W: Effects of Vertebral Axial Decompression on Intradiscal pressure. J Neurosurg, 1994,81:350-353 [Pubmed] [Google Scholar]

9. Tyler Wheeler, MD: Spinal Decompression Therapy.2021 [WebMD]

10. Yang HS: The Effects of Lumbar traction and decompression traction on patients. Dan-Kook University, Dissertation of master's degree, 2008.

CHAPTER 17: HOW THE ACCU-SPINA DECOMPRESSION SYSTEM CAN HELP YOUR BACK PAIN

Accu-Spina is a non-invasive chiropractic device widely used for invertebrate differential dynamics (IDD) disc treatment, which focuses on low back pain caused by compression and degeneration (Schimmel et al., 2009; Wheeler, 2021). Initially developed in the late 1990s, the Accu-Spina decompression system deals with shortcomings associated with traditional traction and limitations of surgical outcomes (Patnaik, 2018). The decompression system involves unloading the spinal discs and facet joints using axial pull or distraction, positioning, and relation to relieve pain related to the discs and increase the spine's functionality. It uses a highly sensitive computer-guided precision to facilitate treatment protocol through variable pressure adjustments.

The Accu-Spina decompression device works by lowering the intradiscal pressure, which enables retraction and repositioning of the compressed disc (also called herniated, prolapsed, ruptured, slipped, or bulging discs). The compressed disc is the root cause of various problems affecting the neck and back. Additionally, the decompression effect causes the accumulation of nutrients in the degenerative disc, which enhances recovery. The Accu-Spina decompression system is a European Conformity (CE) and Class II Food and Drug Administration (FDA) approved medical device, licensed for IDD disc treatment (Patnaik, 2018). However, IDD therapy contains varying traction sessions tailored for specific patients that could take 25-30 therapeutic sessions (Ezinne et al., 2021). A special treatment for each individual is created by a computer using patient-specific information. The device has achieved a significant status among major accomplishments in medical innovation. For this reason, the equipment has been archived at the International Museum of Surgical Science in Chicago, the U.S., for posterity.

Accu-Spina Decompression System Vs. Tradition Traction Systems

The Accu-Spina is a high-tech medical device with a significant success rate for non-surgical lower back and necks spinal compared to traditional traction systems. The Accu-Spina decompression system uses a highly integrated software program that allows the physicians to track the distraction forces applied to a particular injured disc segment, thereby giving real-time patient response (Patnaik, 2018). Compared to traction decompression systems, which distribute the pull of weights in disc sections, thus reducing the pull force required to relieve disc pressure, the Accu-Spina isolates disc problems precisely using distinctive distraction angles (pull), which helps lower the pressure within each segment (Patnaik, 2018). The special angle of pull in the Accu-Spina decompression system eliminates the potential reaction of nearby muscles, unlike traction systems which cause adjacent muscles to spasm due to increased pressure on the discs (Patnaik, 2018). Unlike most traction devices which use cable and pulley systems, the Accu-Spina uses electric and ultrasound stimulation. The Accu-Spina is also the first decompression medical device to receive two consecutive FDA approvals as Class II Medical Device with 510(k) listing (Kanji & Menhinick, 2017). In terms of success rate, extensive clinical studies have shown that Accu-Spina is the safest and most effective in treating degenerative disc disease than other decompression systems (Nujhat, 2013). Compared to traditional traction with no benefit of scanning, the Accu-Spina decompression system also uses an MRI scan to determine contradictions and help diagnose and set up the treatment plan (Patnaik, 2018).

The Accu-Spina Decompression System is Superior to Other Decompression Systems

The unique technology in the Accu-Spina decompression system makes it superior to other decompression options in the market. The medical device utilizes three distinctive patent waveforms used in various treatment protocols: triangular, square, and sinusoidal (Patnaik, 2018). The computer-guided device has a set of different parameters that are individualized according to specific treatment goals and outcomes, including progression time, regression time, decompression weight, high hold, low hold, high tension, angulation, amplitude, target level (L4, L5, S1), transition time, and oscillation parameters (Patnaik, 2018). This treatment delivery technique facilitates specific mobilization or pulls targeting the vertebra dysfunctional disc to relieve acute back or neck pain. According to Patnaik (2018), increasing research volume indicates sinusoidal and oscillatory waveforms prevent muscle spasms. Advanced design and multi-parameter promote safety and comfort, an essential component that enhances the IDD treatment above other available options (Schaufele et al., 2011). The couch can be adjusted to tilt at different angles to enable patient comfort while upright boarding (Patnaik, 2018). Nonetheless, the fully automated and computer-guided device works with high precision, allowing modification of therapeutic sessions per the requirements in different treatment protocols. It can also be adjusted in the course of the rehabilitative intervention.

Prevalence of Low Back Pain

According to Aybala Koçak (2017, p.1), low back pain (LBP) entails "discomfort associated with, muscle tension, and rigidity in the regions between the 12th rib and gluteal fold at the proximal thigh." It is a prevalent issue affecting many people and is particularly associated with advancing age (Schimmel et al., 2009; Hoy et al., 2010; Wu et al., 2020). Acute LBP can last for about six weeks), sub-acute (6-12 weeks), and chronic (past 12 weeks) (Aybala Koçak, 2017) and is associated with various risk factors, including age, body height, depressive moods, and occupational posture (Waterman et al., 2012). However, the specific cause of the onset of the low back is still not clear. In general, low back pain is regarded as non-specific. Aybala Koçak (2017) points out that lumbar disc herniation is the main cause of LBP and is associated with degenerative disc compression. Most patients with LBP often respond to conservative treatments such as resting, drug therapy, bracing, epidural injections, exercise, and physical therapy (Aybala Koçak, 2017). The pain usually goes away within a few weeks to months. Chronic LBP usually affects individuals' ability to conduct normal day-to-day activities. It is the leading cause of morbidity and reduced labor force availability due to increased disability among people aged 45 (Hill, 2020). It also results in a substantial economic burden on governments, industries, communities, families, and individuals (Hoy et al., 2010).

Meucci and colleagues (2015) highlight that the prevalence of LBP varies dependent on the age ranges, with individuals aged >50 at higher risk compared to those between ages 18-30 years. This is attributable to the fact that individuals aged <30 years are predisposed to occupational and domestic exposures that impact their vertebra in addition to degeneration of the spine as age progresses (Meucci et al., 2015). Aybala Koçak (2017) and Chawla and Berman (2018) point out that approximately 80% of people living in low-income countries experience LBP at some point in their lives. As cited in Wu et al. (2020), the Global Burden of Disease (GBD) indicates that the prevalent number of individuals with degenerative spinal conditions has increased over the years, with approximately 377 million in 1990 and 577 million in 2017. The report suggests that the prevalence of LBP has increased from 1.4 -15.5%, while the overall mean incidence has significantly risen from 0.24-7.0% (Fatoye et al., 2019).

Effectiveness of the Accu-Spina Decompression System

The Accu-Spina Decompression System is widely approved by medical regulatory bodies in the United States and globally (Kanji & Menhinick, 2017). Due to its effectiveness, the FDA issued a 510(k) listing clearance under the food, drug, and cosmetics act in section 513(i) (1) (A) of the U.S. Constitution. This suggests that equipment safety is guaranteed to all patients suffering from spinal conditions and that the Decompression System is legally in the market. The device has proved effective in treating an array of vertebra discomfort associated with conditions such as degenerative disc disease and herniated discs. Since its development, clinical reports have documented an impressive success rate of the device in treating lumbar disc problems associated with spinal decompression. Numerous studies also highlight the effectiveness of the Accu-Spina decompression system as a medical device (Kanji & Menhinick, 2017; Ekediegwu and colleagues, 2021). For instance, a retrospective study conducted by Ezinne and colleagues (2005) claimed a 76% decrease in discomfort within a shorter timeframe using the Accu-Spina decompression system on 24 patients with LBP. According to Schimmel et al. (2009), the decompression system reduces low back pain discomfort, thus promoting quality of life. The device can yield positive results with an 85% success rate in patients with lumbar rapture in the vertebral disc, as well as among 76% of participants suffering from facet arthrosis (Schimmel et al., 2009).

Henry (2017), in his evidence-based study seeking to investigate the effectiveness of IDD therapy, also noted that the Accu-Spina decompression system leads to significant improvements in alleviating spinal discomfort. Another study by Kanji and Menhinick (2017) involving 33 patients suffering from lower back pain indicated that subjecting the patients to therapy of 20 traction sessions (entailing pulling the spine) resulted in improved patient outcomes within a few months amongst 76% of the participants with herniated decompression condition. Ekediegwu and colleagues (2021) also noted a significant reduction in chronic BP using NSD in their retrospective pre-post study involving traditional physiotherapy and the Accu-Spina decompression system. The pre-test study conducted by Ekediegwu et al. (2021) assessed 141 adult patients (81 males and 60 females) with a history of discogenic pathology over three years while under routine physiotherapy and treatment using Accu-Spina for an average of 10 sessions over two months noted a significant improvement in low back pain over a short period using the Accu-Spina decompression system compared to other pain relief physiotherapy modalities.

The Expected Timeframe to See Improvement with the Accu-Spina Decompression System

The Accu-Spina treatment modality is rapid and takes a relatively shorter timeframe before patients experience improved mobility and reduced pain due to compression surrounding the injured disc. On average, optimal results are often witnessed within 4-6 weeks of IDD therapy using the decompression system. According to Patnaik (2018), Accu-Spina decompression therapy is achieved through 25 sessions (20 sessions in 10 weeks and five sessions for maintenance over five months) to ensure the long-term success of the treatment. Patient outcomes usually improve between the 5th - 7th sessions. The treatment session lasts for about 25 minutes. Study findings on the efficacy of the Accu-Spina decompression system suggest that early intervention is associated with shorter periods of hospitalization (Wilson et al., 2017). The duration under treatment is determined by the physician depending on the nature of damage to the discs. Typically, corrective chiropractors evaluate the patient's spine thoroughly before initiating NSD therapy. Upon finalizing the diagnosis, the doctor carefully plans the treatment program. A longer recovery time is required for significant damage to the spine.

In most cases, pain from a herniated or bulging disc gets better within days with a positive mental attitude, restricted activity, physical exercise therapy, and taking over-the-counter medications (Hooten, 2013). After initial treatment for a herniated disk, using the Accu-Spina decompression system, the therapists often recommend one to two days of bed rest to help relieve pain and enhance the recovery period. Nonsteroidal anti-inflammatory medications (NSAIDs) such as ibuprofen and naproxen are sometimes prescribed to help relieve pain faster. Nevertheless, engaging in regular light physical exercise such as yoga can help yield immediate optimal results, by strengthening the lower back and abdominal muscles, after IDDT. Ultimately, the results of the Accu-Spina decompression system are generally excellent. Patients tend to experience more improvements from spinal pain within a short period and can resume their normal activities.

The Suggested Frequency of Visits When Using the Accu-Spina Decompression System

Treatment with the Accu-Spina decompression system often requires 20-30 traction sessions to achieve optimal results (Shah et al., 2020). With each session averaging about 45 minutes to one hour in duration, the treatment modality requires patients to make five hospital visits each week for the first two weeks. For additional treatments, the patients are advised to reduce the frequency of visits to three times per week for the remaining few weeks of treatment to achieve the best results. Individualized treatment protocols are usually based on previous results, with each session building on the last therapy. The highly computerized medical device can store large volumes of therapists' data for pathological diagnosis and treatment. As a result, sessions are scheduled one day apart to keep track of the progress. Maintaining a positive attitude is critical for healing, and doctors always emphasize the importance of compliance with the IDD therapy protocols.

In their randomized control trial, Kanji and Menhinick (2017) subjected the study participants (IDD and SHAM groups) to 20 sessions using the Accu-Spina decompression system, according to the IDD Therapy protocol. The program also consisted of a one-hour training duration two times per week during the 12 weeks study period.

The IDD Therapy protocol has been developed over the years following multiple simulations and has been tested on thousands of patients with high success rates. Therefore, therapists recommend that patients adhere to treatment schedules to achieve positive health outcomes.

Contraindications to Using the Accu-Spina Decompression System

There is limited scientific evidence suggesting contraindications of utilizing the Accu-Spina decompression system to treat neck and back pain. Multiple results from clinical trials indicate that patients rarely get complications from using the treatment modality. Moreover, many studies and clinical trials have shown that Accu-Spina is highly effective in treating various spinal conditions despite some contradictions. Like any other medical procedure, the decompression system comes with a set of risk factors as it is a minimally invasive procedure. Considering the risk of pressure on the abdomen, the Accu-Spina Decompression System is not recommended for pregnant women (Soltani, 2019). Increased uterine size might occur due to expansion by distension and mechanical stretching of the muscle fibers caused by waveforms produced by the machine. The decompression system can also have adverse effects on patients with spinal instability or recovering from spinal surgery due to interference with implanted screws or metal plates (Pingel & Kandziora, 2013). Increasing research shows that the intervention to chronic back pain using non-surgical decompression techniques can enhance the spread of metastatic cancer to the bones (Kurisunkal et al., 2020).

A follow-up MRI study conducted by Gil and colleagues (2021) indicates that unlike surgical decompression treatment modality, which can identify disc space infections, the Accu-Spina can potentially worsen the condition because it involves non-invasive procedures. Other conditions that may worsen with the use of the decompression system include patients with severe nerve damage, aortic aneurysm, and enhanced spondylolisthesis (non-aligned sections of the vertebra) (Gil et al.,2021). To prevent these potential risks, chiropractic doctors usually recommend patients to undergo multiple screening tests, including a physical exam, MRI, and X-Rays to establish whether non-surgical decompression systems are applicable for treatment. Despite these limitations, decompression traction using Accu-Spina has yielded highly successful results in treating multiple vertebra conditions. In their prospective comprehensive cohort study, Kim et al. (2021) suggest that non-surgical spinal treatment results in less patient outcome compared to surgical decompression, which is effective in the short term. However, significant results using the NSD usually have a long-term impact.

Overall Benefits of the Accu-Spina Decompression System

Based on the information above, it is evident that the Accu-Spina decompression system has various advantages in treating low back pain. These advantages include:

a. *It is safe and cost-effective*: Unlike surgical decompression, which is associated with tissue damage, excessive bleeding, and infection at the operation site, the Accu-Spina decompression device is non-invasive, making it a safer treatment option. Compared to other non-surgical decompression systems, the Accu-Spina decompression system's motorized traction poses a limited risk of spasm to adjacent muscles due to increased pressure on the discs. The machine's enhanced safety is also attributed to multi-parameters incorporated in the computerized system, allowing tracking of therapy progress and increasing precision. In addition, the device is approved by the FDA and CE to deliver IDD treatment.

b. *It is superior to traditional traction*: Unlike traditional traction techniques, which are often non-precise, the Accu-Spina decompression technology can distract and mobilize specific spine segments, thereby decompressing the targeted intervertebral disc. Controlled forces can safely work on the para-spinal tissues with significant pressure differentials without causing muscle spasms. Moreover, most traction devices use cable and pulley systems, while the Accu-Spina uses electric and ultrasound stimulation. The Accu-Spina decompression system also uses an MRI scan to determine contradictions and help diagnose and set up the treatment plan, which is unavailable in the traditional traction system.

c. *It is better than other decompression systems available on the market:* The unique technology in the Accu-Spina decompression system uses three distinctive patent waveforms used in various treatment protocols: triangular, square, and sinusoidal. As a result, it enables specific mobilization or pulls targeting the vertebra dysfunctional disc to relieve acute back or neck pain. The Accu-Spina decompression device uses sinusoidal force to replace the linear distraction forces, promoting excellent safety and comfort. This eliminates the risk of the patient undergoing spasms, which may elevate intradiscal pressure and pain. The sinusoidal waveform also enables oscillatory forces, thereby mobilizing the joint in a longitudinal plane instead of the anterior-posterior plane at the targeted disc. Additionally, the fully automated and computer-guided device allows therapeutic sessions to be modified as needed in various treatment protocols and adjusted during the rehabilitative intervention.

d. ***It is highly effective.*** According to multiple clinical trials, pilot studies, and evidence-based practice, the innovation has a success rate of 86-91%, with many patients reporting significant relief within a short timeframe. The decompression system effectively treats severe conditions like degenerative disc disease and posterior facet disorder.

e. ***It is comfortable:*** The Accu-Spina decompression table promotes safety and comfort, thus enhancing IDD therapy outcomes. The couch can be adjusted to tilt at different angles to enable patient comfort during upright boarding.

f. ***It is rapid and takes a relatively shorter timeframe to show improved outcomes***: The optimal results are often observed within 4-6 weeks of the therapy using the Accu-Spina decompression system. Patient outcomes usually improve between the 5th- 7th sessions. The prementioned studies indicate that the Accu-Spina decompression system is associated with reduced hospitalizations. The Accu-Spina decompression system often requires 20-30 traction sessions to achieve optimal results, with each session averaging about 45 minutes to one hour in duration. The treatment modality requires patients to make hospital visits five times a week for the first two weeks. In the rest of the sessions, patients are advised to reduce the frequency of visits to three times per week for the remaining few weeks of treatment to achieve the best results.

g. ***It has minimal contradictions:*** Research indicates that patients rarely get complications from using the treatment modality. Moreover, many research studies and clinical trials have shown that Accu-Spina is highly effective in treating various spinal conditions despite some contradictions.

Conclusion

With the increased prevalence of lower back pain, mainly due to advancing age, the Accu-Spina traction table has gained a cutting edge over other treatment options. Overall, the decompression system effectively treats severe vertebral conditions like degenerative disc disease and posterior facet disorder. Its unique and advanced technology makes the medical equipment superior to other decompression options in the market. Unlike traditional traction decompression systems, the Accu-Spina utilizes a highly integrated software program that allows therapists to track the forces applied to injured discs, giving the real-time patient response. The distinctive patent waveforms (triangular, square, and sinusoidal) reduce the potential for muscle spasms. Nonetheless, the traction table advanced design also promotes safety and comfort, thus enhancing IDD Therapy outcomes. As outlined in various scientific evidence from clinical trials, the Accu-Spina has a significant success rate of 86-91%. The equipment is also compliant with European Conformity (CE) and approved as a Class II medical device by the Food and Drug Administration (FDA).

Evidence-based study results pertaining to the efficacy of the Accu-Spina decompression system indicate that patients usually experience improved mobility and reduced pain within a shorter period of intervention. Averagely, optimal results can be achieved within 4-6 weeks of IDD therapy using the decompression system. Typically, chronic back and neck pain treatment using the Accu-Spina follows the IDD Therapy protocol of about 20-30 sessions, each averaging 45 minutes to 1hr. The treatment modality requires patients to make hospital visits five times a week for the first two weeks. Although the Accu-Spina has its shortcoming, such as restricted use on pregnant women, individuals with implanted screws or metal plates, and those with spinal instability, the equipment's success rate in terms of the improved outcome makes it superior to other decompression systems. However, more research should be conducted to bridge the knowledge gap by providing more scientific evidence.

References

1. Aybala Koçak, F. (2017). Comparison of the short-term effects of the conventional motorized traction with non-surgical spinal decompression performed with a DRX9000TM device on pain, functionality, depression, and quality of life in patients with low back pain associated with lumbar disc herniation: A single-blind randomized controlled trial. *Turkish Journal of Physical Medicine and Rehabilitation, 64*(1), 17-27. https://doi.org/10.5606/tftrd.2017.154

2. Chawla, J., & Berman, S. (2018). *What is the prevalence of low back pain (LBP)?* Medscape.com. Retrieved 22 October 2021, from https://www.medscape.com/answers/1144130-118907/what-is-the-prevalence-of-low-back-pain-lbp.

3. Ekediegwu, E., Chuka, C., Nwosu, I., Ogbueche, C., Ekechukwu, E. N. D., Uchenwoke, C., & Odole, A. (2021). *Musculoskeletal Disorders and Treatment.*

4. Ezinne, E., Chike, C., Chigozie, U., Ifeoma, N., & Adesola, O. (2005). Reduction in Chronic Low Back Pain Using Intervertebral Differential Dynamics Therapy (IDDT) and Routine Physiotherapy: A Retrospective Pre-Post Study. *Journal of Musculoskeletal Disorders and Treatment, 7*(2). https://doi.org/10.23937/2572-3243.1510098

5. Fatoye, F., Gebrye, T., & Odeyemi, I. (2019). Real-world incidence and prevalence of low back pain using routinely collected data. *Rheumatology International, 39*(4), 619-626. https://doi.org/10.1007/s00296-019-04273-0

6. Gil, H. Y., Choi, E., Jiyoun, J., Han, W. K., Nahm, F. S., & Lee, P. B. (2021). Follow-Up Magnetic Resonance Imaging Study of Non-Surgical Spinal Decompression Therapy for Acute Herniated Intervertebral Disc: A Prospective, Randomized, Controlled Study.

7. Henry, L. (2017). Non-surgical Spinal Decompression an Effective Physiotherapy Modality for Neck and Back Pain. *Journal of Novel Physiotherapy and Physical Rehabilitation,* 4(3), 062-065.

8. Hill, J. (2020). *Patients pay thousands for back pain treatment — with little scientific evidence that it works.* NBC News. Retrieved 23 October 2021, from https://www.nbcnews.com/news/us-news/patients-pay-thousands-back-pain-treatment-little-scientific-evidence-it-n1247993.

9. Hooten, W. M., Timming, R., Belgrade, M., Gaul, J., Goertz, M., Haake, B., ... & Walker, N. (2013). Assessment and

management of chronic pain. *Institute for Clinical Systems Improvement*, 106.

10. Hoy, D., Brooks, P., Blyth, F., & Buchbinder, R. (2010). The Epidemiology of low back pain. *Best Practice & Research Clinical Rheumatology*, *24*(6), 769-781. https://doi.org/10.1016/j.berh.2010.10.002

11. Kanji, G., & Menhinick, P. (2017). No effect of traction in patients with low back pain: A single-center, single-blind, randomized controlled trial of Intervertebral Differential Dynamics Therapy.

12. Kim, C. H., Choi, Y., Chung, C. K., Kim, K. J., Shin, D. A., Park, Y. K., ... & Cho, Y. (2021). Non-surgical treatment outcomes for surgical candidates with lumbar disc herniation: a comprehensive cohort study. *Scientific reports*, *11*(1), 1-12.

13. Kurisunkal, V., Gulia, A., & Gupta, S. (2020). Principles of management of spine metastasis. *Indian journal of orthopedics*, *54*(2), 181-193.

14. Meucci, R., Fassa, A., & Faria, N. (2015). Prevalence of chronic low back pain: systematic review. *Revista De Saúde Pública*, *49*(0). https://doi.org/10.1590/s0034-8910.2015049005874

15. Nujhat, M. (2013). *Prevalence of low back pain among the people age over forty at a selected village in Nator* (Doctoral dissertation, Department of Physiotherapy, Bangladesh Health Professions Institute, CRP).

16. Patnaik, G. (2018). Role of IDD Therapy in the Back and Neck Pain. *Journal Of Medicine: Study & Research, 1*(1), 1-5. https://doi.org/10.24966/msr-5657/100002

17. Pingel, A., & Kandziora, F. (2013). Anterior decompression and fusion for cervical spinal canal stenosis. *European Spine Journal, 22*(3), 673.

18. Schaufele, M. K., & Newsome, M. (2011). Intervertebral Differential Dynamics (IDD) Therapy vs. Exercise Based Physical Therapy–Results from a Randomized Controlled Trial. *Physikalische Medizin, Rehabilitationsmedizin, Kurortmedizin, 21*(01), 34-40.

19. Shah, A., Sheth, M. S., & Shah, D. A. (2020). Effect of non-surgical spinal decompression therapy on walking duration in subjects with lumbar radiculopathy: A randomized controlled trial. *International Journal of Medical Science and Public Health, 9*(8).

20. Schimmel, J., de Kleuver, M., Horsting, P., Spruit, M., Jacobs, W., & van Limbeek, J. (2009). No effect of traction in patients with low back pain: a single centre, single-blind, randomized controlled trial of Intervertebral Differential Dynamics Therapy®. *European Spine Journal, 18*(12), 1843-1850. https://doi.org/10.1007/s00586-009-1044-3

21. Soltani, S., Nogaro, M. C., Kieser, S. C. J., Wyatt, M. C., & Kieser, D. C. (2019). Spontaneous spinal epidural hematomas in pregnancy: a systematic review. *World neurosurgery, 128*, 254-258.

22. Waterman, B., Belmont, P., & Schoenfeld, A. (2012). Low back pain in the United States: incidence and risk factors for presentation in the emergency setting. *The Spine Journal, 12*(1), 63-70. https://doi.org/10.1016/j.spinee.2011.09.002

23. Wilson, J. R., Tetreault, L. A., Kwon, B. K., Arnold, P. M., Mroz, T. E., Shaffrey, C., ... & Fehlings, M. G. (2017). Timing of decompression in patients with acute spinal cord injury: a systematic review. *Global spine journal*, 7(3_suppl), 95S-115S.

24. Wu, A., March, L., Zheng, X., Huang, J., Wang, X., & Zhao, J. et al. (2020). Global low back pain prevalence and years lived with disability from 1990 to 2017: estimates from the Global Burden of Disease Study 2017. *Annals Of Translational Medicine, 8*(6), 299-299. https://doi.org/10.21037/atm.2020.02.175

CHAPTER 18: THE POWER OF RED LIGHT THERAPY

Red light therapy, also known as photo rejuvenation, is a technology that uses visible red light wavelengths from 630-660 nanometers and infrared light wavelengths at 880nm to penetrate deep into the layers of the skin where they increase energy inside cells as well as stimulate the production of collagen and elastin. Skin layers, because of their high content of blood and water, absorb light very readily. Photo rejuvenation has become recognized as one of the safest, quickest, and most affordable ways to make dramatic anti-aging changes in the skin.

Red light therapy involves having low-power red light wavelengths emitted directly through the skin, although this process cannot be felt and isn't painful because it doesn't produce any heat. Red light can be absorbed into the skin to a depth of about eight to 10 millimeters, at which point it has positive effects on cellular energy and multiple nervous systems and metabolic processes.

Light therapy in different forms has been around for ages. In fact, the ancient Greek doctor, Hippocrates, was known to counsel patients on the benefits of light and recommended that they expose themselves to sunlight to treat various health conditions. In more recent times NAS, while doing plant growth experiments in outer space, discovered that red and infrared LEDs (light emitting diodes) healed injuries at a much faster pace. Since those discoveries, light has been harnessed and studied fervently revealing countless benefits and therapeutic uses.

Fast forward to today, and you will find red light therapy in dermatologist offices, chiropractor offices, physicians, spas, clinics, salons, and in the home. As this therapy gains popularity, some may be a bit skeptical and asking whether or not this therapy does work.

The straightforward answer is a resounding yes!

When Was Red Light Therapy Was Discovered?

Light therapy is something that has been going on for several thousand years. The LED light technology was originally developed for NASA plant growth experiments and was found to be helpful in speeding up healing in outer space. Doctors began to experiment with LEDs for the treatment of wounds in hospitals where they discovered that red and infrared LEDs increase the energy inside cells and boost the activity of mitochondria (the powerhouse in cells.)

It was found that some skin cells may grow 150-200 percent faster when exposed to LEDs which speeds up the healing and reparative processes so the skin and body can repair past and current damage. The ancient Greeks actually used it. They knew that sunlight was good for your health. They did not know about vitamin D and the benefits it has for the skin and the body, although they could see how sunlight benefited them.

In 1903, a scientist of Icelandic descent, Niels Finsen, was awarded the Nobel Prize in medicine in recognition of his discovery that light therapy could help treat certain diseases, such as lupus, opening a new area of research. He showed that phototherapy, certain wavelengths of light, could have beneficial medical effects.

Since then, light therapy has been a focus of research more in Eastern Europe, Russia, and Japan than the United States. Russian researchers have published hundreds of studies on the benefits of light therapy, but few have been translated into English. The research showed that such therapy has significant healing effects on human tissue.

How Long Does The Treatment Last?

The Red Light Therapy is not an immediate miracle transformation that will occur overnight, but it will provide you with ongoing improvements that you will begin to see in anywhere from 24 hours to 2 months, depending on the condition, its severity, and how regularly the light is used.

There are few immediate changes to the skin, as change occurs naturally for weeks. Everyone reacts differently, depending on their age and the condition of their skin. In general, best results are achieved over an 8 – 12 week period.

So whether you are using an infrared heating pad, a 2-panel LED device or single heat lamp therapy – It will depend on the extent of the pain and your health condition. Some will use infrared light for pain once and feel immediate results (which can last for more than 6 hours), while others will have to use the system 2 to 3 times in a row before they feel significant pain relief.

How Does Red Light Therapy Work?

Red light therapy is a form of phototherapy, which involved being exposed to daylight or specific wavelengths of light using various light sources dependent on the clinical indication. The light exposure is prescribed for a particular length of time, and occasional doses must be given at certain times of the day. Red light therapy penetrates deeper into the skin than other light wavelengths and is thought to rejuvenate skin.

When red light penetrates the skin, it powers up the natural healing properties of our body at a cellular level. The light stimulates blood circulation which also results in increased lymphatic system activity that promotes draining of interstitial fluid from tissues and transports white blood cells to areas where it is needed. Because of this, it activates our body's metabolic processes and spurs the creation of collagen and fibroblasts. It also increases cellular clean up to reduce inflammation.

Red light therapy is the process of exposing skin to red light wavelengths which have low energy. Unlike other light wavelengths, this is absorbed into the skin to a depth of about 10mm where it can heat and positively affect cells and processes within the body. Different wavelengths of light can be used to target the skin differently and treat varying conditions. There are virtually no adverse effects of red light therapy and can have many benefits.

Red light therapy has been proven to effectively treat skin issues such as; fine lines, wrinkles, large pores, rough skin, and crow's feet. Red light therapy effectively and gently makes significant changes in the skin at a deep level repairing cells, collagen, and elastin.

Light emitting diodes (LEDs) produce wavelengths which are measured in nanometers. The higher the nanometer number, the longer the wavelength and the deeper the light penetrates into the body. Specific nanometer ranges have been researched and shown to penetrate into skin, tissue, joints, and bones where the light is then absorbed at a cellular level. Once absorbed, the healing wavelengths prompt over 24 positive reactions, including:

- Boosting circulation
- Increasing collagen and elastin synthesis
- Sparking cellular energy (ATP)
- Encouraging healing and reparative processes to engage
- Increase the production of endorphins
- Block pain-transmitting neurons

As these reactions begin to occur within the cells and tissues, changes ensue within the skin and body.

Are Their Negative Side Effects Of Red Light Therapy?

Red light therapy is considered to be a safe and well-tolerated therapy for the relief of symptoms of multiple conditions. Light therapy that involves only visible light is generally considered safe. Still, negative effects may occur. As a consequence of light therapy, patients can complain of irritability, headaches, eye strain, sleep disturbances, and insomnia. Mild visual side effects are not unusual but remit promptly. Therefore determining the appropriate dose and timing of light is essential to diminish the occurrence of such side effects.

The use of phototherapy for people with drug-resistant non-seasonal depression can result in a hyperactive state called mania. In these rare cases light therapy must be reduced or stopped and the condition adequately treated. Also, any treatment where the patient is exposed to ultraviolet radiation is not entirely without its risks – including premature aging of the skin and an increased possibility for skin cancer development later in life. Eye strain and temporary headaches caused by the light are also often reported, although these symptoms do not seem to indicate any permanent injury.

The most common risk associated with this therapy is shining it in your eyes. Not that red or infrared light itself is damaging to your eyes, but the devices can produce high glare. Reputable products will come with eye protection, and it should be worn during every facial treatment. If you are using the light for non-facial applications, such as wound care or pain relief, just be careful to not to shine the light in your eyes. (The same goes for your pets.) Never look directly into the red light therapy device.

What Are The Signs That Would Indicate That Red Light Therapy Is Effective?

Red light therapy is not only extremely beneficial in the fight against aging but does not harm the skin like lasers can. It is safe for all skin types, non-invasive, non-ablative (skin damaging), no downtime, no pain, and simple. The wavelengths gently penetrate and promote healthy skin, tissue, and cells without causing any harm. LED light therapy is one of the few non-invasive tools available that can actually reverse the signs of aging.

Red light therapy has been shown to be effective for the treatment of pain, relief of muscle and joint aches, sprains, and back pain. Red light and infrared light wavelengths penetrate deep into the body easing pain and repairing damaged tissue. Infrared light at 880nm penetrates to a depth of about 30-40 mm which makes it very effective for bones, joints, and deep muscle problems. Red light at 660nm penetrates to a depth of about 8-10mm which makes it beneficial for treating problems closer to the surface of the skin such as wounds, cuts, scars, and infection.

Also, a ground-breaking study has just recently shown that light therapy has the ability to improve cognitive function after traumatic brain injury. At home, daily light therapy treatments when placed on the forehead and scalp have been shown to make dramatic improvements in cognitive function including improved memory, inhibition, and the ability to sustain attention and focus.

How Often Should A Patient Be Treated With Red Light Therapy To See Results?

Every individual may respond differently to specific treatments and results will also depend on the goal you want to achieve. Everyone reacts differently, depending on their age and the condition of their skin. In general, best results are achieved over an 8 – 12 week period.

It is important to take before and after pictures to document your progress. Results will be subtle, and it is important to set your expectations right. This is not magic, and the results do not show overnight. However, with daily use, you should be able to see improvements in 4 to 6 weeks.

Also, it is recommended to start with a commitment of 15 minutes, which is the maximum time in our Red Light Therapy bed, at least 3-5 times per week for the first 1-4 weeks. Then you should use the Red Light Therapy bed at least 2-3 times per week for the following 4-12 weeks, and finally 1-2 times per week to maintain your desired skin results.

Does Red Light Therapy Reduce Pain Immediately?

The red light of a particular wavelength can penetrate into cells, and as their wavelength matches with skin tissue, the water or blood cannot block the red light waves. The light has therapeutic effects which promote faster healing of wounds, heals burns, muscle, and joint pain. The device utilizes the ability of the skin to absorb light of a particular wavelength and to convert it into cellular energy and promote the natural healing of tissue.

In the case of any unusual redness or inflammation after using the device, you immediately need to stop using it and consult your doctor. When you use a light therapy device at home, you need to be careful so as not to expose your eyes to the light. You can also use protective eye pads to protect your eyes from exposure to red light.

What Are The Forms Of Light Therapy?

The most common type of light therapy is of course also the most common source of light - the sun. This sort of therapy has been around for millennia. The most obvious therapeutic effect comes from the UV spectrum contained in sunlight. UV rays are deadly to almost all microorganisms which might attack all superficial wounds. The infrared portion of sunlight (heat) increases circulation and metabolic activity of the area which it hits. Here are some major forms of light therapy:

Infrared Light Therapy

It involves the use of infrared radiation emitted from heat lamps. They are devices that radiate heat to stimulate different biological effects like increased oxygen usage and enzymatic rates as well as dissociation. It is a procedure that is painless and non-invasive.

Blue Light Therapy

This is another type of phototherapy that is non-invasive, FDA-approved, and used for treating acne vulgaris or kill off bacteria on your skin. It is a procedure that can be carried out inside the office of a dermatologist.

Ultraviolet Radiation

This form of therapy came after the heat lamps. It was considered a major breakthrough because by simply switching on a UV light bulb, a wound or sample of blood could be sterilized of any unwanted organisms or chemicals. Also, stabilization of protein changes became possible with different wavelengths of UV light, allowing for longer storage of plasma in blood banks. Once again there are varying wavelengths of UV radiation.

Light Amplification by Stimulated Emission of Radiation (L.A.S.E.R.)

Lasers are still considered by many medical professionals to be one of the hallmarks of modern medicine. They produce very precise and intense pulses of photons and deliver them to a target. On the electromagnetic spectrum, wavelengths are measured in nanometers (one billionth of a meter). An individual laser contains photons of only one color. That means that a laser operates at only a single frequency or wavelength.

Is There Any Research On The Benefits Of Red Light Therapy?

The main benefits of red light therapy are thought to have come from the energy exchange. The responses of cells and tissues to red light therapy, which does not itself produce much heat, can be comparable to the body's reaction to heat. The red light therapy can be used for serious medical treatment, reducing inflammation and pain in your body. For those who suffer pain from broken bones, torn muscles, tendonitis, strains, sprains, arthritis, and fibromyalgia, this therapy becomes one alternative for drug treatment. This is ideal for those who don't like taking drug for medical treatment. Here are the major benefits of red light therapy

Better Circulation and Collagen Production

When the light penetrates through the epidermal and dermal skin layers, it increases circulation to help form new capillaries. It also increases collagen production and fibroblasts. Red therapy light improves collagen levels naturally by triggering the body to produce more of its own. Increased collagen doesn't just give the skin a wrinkle-free glow, but its ability to improve joint health makes it great for people living with arthritis. It can be helpful for those with a variety of painful musculoskeletal issues.

Aids Pain Relief

The reduction in pain relief can come from a combination of the above effects on tissues. Joint stiffness, muscle spasms, restricted blood flow, and inflammation can all cause and contribute to pain. By reducing those symptoms, red light therapy can, therefore, reduce pain.

Improves Elasticity of Collagen Fibres

Red light therapy at certain wavelengths is thought to stimulate the productions of collagen and elastin fibers, as well as the creation of new capillaries. A greater number of capillaries within the skin will improve blood flow to the skin tissues and therefore the transportation of oxygen and nutrients to the cells, while the extra collagen and elastin will smooth and plump-out the skin. This can slow and reduce the effects of aging on the skin, giving a more youthful appearance.

Supports Detoxification and Circulation

Photobiomodulation stimulates an increase in lymphatic system activity, which as discussed in this post on dry brushing assists with detoxification. It also increases circulation via the formation of new capillaries, allowing more blood and oxygen to deliver nutrients throughout the body

Hair Growth, Thickness, and Shine

No, it won't cause you to grow hair in new places (whew!), but several studies have found that red light therapy can increase hair follicle activity. For example, in this analysis, hair thickness, density, and shine were improved with light therapy.

Help for the Thyroid and Hormones

Researchers have found that it also has a beneficial impact on thyroid function for both women and men. There is also some evidence to suggest it may increase testosterone production in men.

Recover Faster from Injury and Illness

Red light therapy increases circulation and ATP production throughout the body which may help speed healing during times of illness. It also stimulates lymph system activity and phagocytosis, the process of cells cleaning house.

CHAPTER 19: HOW THE NEUROMED SYSTEM CAN HELP YOUR BACK PAIN

Pain has become one of the most common problems worldwide. It leads a patient to consult a physician. Research has shown that more than 40 million people undergo musculoskeletal pain. And more than 300 million physician visits end up costing millions and billions of dollars annually. Low back pain is one of the leading causes of physical pain in the United States. It is more probable among older. However, it is common that lead to disability under 45 years old.

Coping with pain is not as convenient as it seems. There is an immediate need to relieve pain to let the patients live better and more satisfying lives. It is somehow possible with the help of pain medications. However, the effect to relieve pain is just temporary with undesirable side effects. Therefore, FDA has approved NeuroMed Electroanalgesic Delivery System, a medical device, that assists in order to stimulating the peripheral nerve to relieve pain. It may help provide symptomatic relief of chronic long-term pain.

History

Science has come a long way in advancement. Evidence investigated electrical stimulation has treated several medical conditions successfully for around 2,000 years. There was a medical doctor in ancient Greece who reported the application of electromedicine for the very first time. Largus and Dioscorides, great physicians, explored relieving gout pain by electric ray in a foot bath. These electrical impulses are utilized to treat circulation disorders and pain. The pain arising from severe headaches, neuralgia, and arthritis was limited by the electrotherapy shocks championed by Largus and Dioscorides. It has been analyzed by Benjamin franklin during this whole time that electric shock may contribute to relieving pain from a frozen shoulder.

Later by 1800, more than 50% of American physicians utilized different kinds of electro medicines for wound healing and pain management. In 1910, the use of electromedicine was declined in the physician's private practice due to a misleading report. This report devalued electromedicine in the human body. However, it got recognition again in 1950 when in Germany, a medical company developed better electrical devices. The purpose of these devices was to enable medical treatments to the human skin that were safely delivered to deep tissue.

Medical and healthcare professionals then used interferential current worldwide. Later, a Gate Control Theory helped in validating electromedical treatment, TENS. It is known as Transcutaneous Electric Nerve Stimulation. It is associated with portable battery-operated devices. Their electrodes are strapped at the pain site. It eventually applies a current that works in relieving pain (Braun, *et al*, 2021).

Nowadays, NeuroMed Electroanalgesia treatment is widely used by American physicians that give shocks to the depth of tissue and reduce pain instantly. It helps in circulatory conditions. It has been assessed that only the last 15 years were enough to get recognition for these valuable treatments for pain management. It has become renowned and preferred over drug therapy. Because drug therapy is costly and has side effects that cause irritation to your body. Also, Electroanalgesia is preferred over surgery. Surgeries are also known for their high cost, invasive, and chances of ineffectiveness. This is how NeuroMed Electroanalegsia (EA) has evolved and become valuable around the globe.

Introduction

You must be curious to know more about NeuroMed, which provides long-term pain relief. Basically, Electroanalgesia (EA) is drug-free, non-surgical, and highly effective. NeuroMed is an efficient pain management system that delivers accurate dosages of electrical stimulation to the nerves connecting the brain and spinal cord to organs and limbs. These nerves are known as peripheral nerves. This alternative approach to relieving pain does not just stimulate nerves but also helps in enhancing local blood circulation. It is highly effective in managing symptomatic relief of chronic pain (long-term). Neuromed has made life easier for surgeons to do neurologic procedures and reduce their patients' pain (Stantun-Hicks, *et al,* 2009).

NeuroMed has to get relief from utilizing highly addictive pharmacotherapy drugs that lead to undesired side effects. This chemical addiction became the main concern of the physicians, which is now completely finished with the widely used NeuroMed Electroanalgesia treatment. Physicians had to give high dosage drugs in order to relieve pain that caused severe dizziness and addiction later. The study analyzes that month-long dosages of pharmaceutical drugs tend to cause severe brain changes. These highly addictive painkillers include Oxycontin, Vicodin, and Percocet. Therefore, it is safe and convenient to use NeuroMed Electroanalgesia treatment without compromising patients' health. This treatment is non-invasive, promising, and effective and instantly facilitates pain management.

This drug-free method effectively promotes healing even in cases that are not supported by epidurals, medications, or even surgery. The time of treatment lies between 15 to 25 minutes. During this whole time, the treatment continues to work on the nerves with the electrical pulses. The resulting time is not so far away, because you see a rapid relief in pain right after this treatment. It leads to improve further within a few minutes. The treated area may feel muscle tension and a tingling sensation for a time. In some cases, patients may undergo mild headaches and fatigued sensation. However, these sensations may disappear over time.

Even after a single treatment, you may feel a notable reduction in pain. However, physicians may need to execute Matrix Electroanalgesia several times in order to get the best possible outcomes. The precise number of treatments varies from person to person as it is based on the pain's severity. Generally, 5 to 15 treatments are expected for the best results.

How does it work?

Those who have undergone physical therapy must know about Transcutaneous Electric Nerve Stimulation (TENS). This is an external device that works by applying low voltage electricity via electrodes that helps lowering pain. These electrodes are placed all over the skin (Dissanayake, *et al*, 2010). Similarly, EA treatment by NeuroMed reduces pain by utilizing electrical frequencies. The difference between TENS and Electroanalgesic (EA) treatment is the rates in EA are much higher than in TENS. For instance, TENS is inclined to deliver 1 to 250 pulses per second. However, 8,300 to 10,000 pulses per second are delivered by EA.

In EA, the electrical energy delivered goes deeper into the tissue of patients. These higher frequencies are more likely to lower the ability of affected nerves to transmit pain signals. Hence, it is inclined to boost healing while reducing pain.

This system is pretty safer when it is delivered with the appropriate dosages and electrodes. The intensity of pain in the patients is reduced effectively. Thus, improving the quality of living for the patients.

This treatment, Electroanalgesia (EA) therapy, utilizes the application of frequency from .1- .5 Hz (physical medicine treatment). It utilizes frequency from 5000 Hz to 8,300 Hz in order to achieve pain relief goals by providing therapeutic action for inflammation, reducing edema, and analgesia, and supporting metabolism in the neuropathic extremity.

How it works is it needs specifically designed conductive sock or hand garment electrodes that are placed all over the treatment area in order to execute Electroanalgesia (EA). It provides a depolarization effect on the nerve cells in order to enhance the healing effect by reducing the ability of affected nerves to transmit pain signals. Particular patented pre-programmed software algorithms are used by this medical device to trigger desired physiological mechanisms of action bio-electrically from frequencies beginning at .1 Hz – .5 Hz (for stimulation). It is required to change the frequencies throughout the therapy to include a 5,000 Hz frequency (Ranu, *et al,* 2011).

80%A High Definition frequency generator (HDfg)™ is used by this technology that has the tendency to produce higher frequencies such as 8,300 Hz for inhibiting the nerves. This EA technology continues to utilize a particular carrier frequency. It is also required that the physician modifies the dosage and intensity to match the parameters accurately. It has been estimated that 75-80% of patients have positive results after utilizing this treatment. The study shows lasting results through the treatment. It is usually successful. However, research shows that 20 to 25% of patients experience a very short-term relief. In such cases, more treatments need to be included to get complete relief from pain.

Conditions Treated by NeuroMed- EA

Neuropathy in Eustis is a dysfunction or disease of one or more peripheral nerves. It usually is a disease of those nerves that branch out through fingers, legs, toes, or arms. It generally leads to tingling, burning, weakness, painful sensation, or numbness. It has been estimated that more than 20 million people undergo some kind of neuropathy. One of the most prevalent causes of neuropathy includes diabetes. Additionally, toxic trauma such as environmental toxins, chemotherapy, or drugs may arise from peripheral neuropathy. It may also be emerged from biomechanical injury, including carpal tunnel syndrome. Placing constant pressure on the nerves may also lead to peripheral neuropathy. Symptoms of peripheral neuropathy include dizziness, imbalance, swollen feet, loss of muscle tone, pain while walking, and changes in gait. Poor nutrition may also worsen the nervous system. If you feel any of such symptoms, you may need

NeuroMed EA. When it comes to its treatment, the goal is to ensure that the bodies' nerves of the patients perform optimally. The purpose is to allow the nervous system to transmit all the messages through the nerves successfully. It is how a patient is able to live a happy and normal life. Matrix Electroanalgesia stimulation therapy is one of the leading therapies that contribute to the cure. In NeuroMed, electro-analgesics are utilized in order to treat neuropathic pain. It also helps patients get rid of medications like Tegretol, Gabapentin, Lyrica, and Neurontin that have adverse effects. NeuroMed technology is used as a non-invasive approach that helps to get relief from nerve damage, pain from neuropathies, and circulation issues. From back pain, bulging discs, and foot pain to fibromyalgia, neck pain, sciatica, and shoulder pain, NeuroMed is effective in relieving all kinds of pain without medications (Liem, *et al,* 2015).

NeuroMed help treat

- Pain arising from neuropathies
- Circulation issues by promoting local blood circulation
- Back pain
- Foot pain and shoulder pain
- Pain associated with sciatica
- Fibromyalgia
- Improve balance and give relief from pain by walking

Contraindications

A few contraindications may include thrombophlebitis, manifest thrombosis, the acute danger of hemorrhage, cardiac demand pacemaker, and disturbances in cardiac rhythm. It is suggested not to stimulate the carotid sinus. Essentially, precautions should be used in patients who have a risk or suspicion of heart problems. Additionally, patients with higher intensity transthoracic applications or epilepsy should be analyzed accordingly.

Final Thoughts on NeuroMed

NeuroMed Electroanalgesia (EA) treatment is a safe, non-toxic, and effective therapy with minimal side effects. In most cases, it results in high satisfaction and compliance, even in critical patients. Basically, this treatment is used to relieve pain in the long term by releasing endorphins in the central nervous system. Endorphins are substances that are known as neuropeptide pain relief. It usually happens in the body. They are enhanced by EA treatment which eventually contributes to relieving long-term pain.

It has been analyzed that Electroanalgesia treatment is considered valuable by renowned physicians. Sometimes, this alone therapy seems to be ineffective, addictive, and costly. Yet, this treatment is investigated by several medical researchers around the globe. They are trying to utilize EA medical treatment in order to treat pain associated with fibromyalgia, carpal tunnel syndrome pain, sciatica pain, or other chronic or acute disorders. It is to provide comfort to the patients.

References

1. Braun, R. G., & Wittenberg, G. F. (2021, March). Motor recovery: how rehabilitation techniques and technologies can enhance recovery and neuroplasticity. In *Seminars in neurology*. Thieme Medical Publishers, Inc..

2. Stanton-Hicks, M. (2009). Peripheral nerve stimulation for pain peripheral neuralgia and complex regional pain syndrome. In *Neuromodulation* (pp. 397-407). Academic Press.

3. Dissanayake, T. D., Budgett, D. M., Hu, P., Bennet, L., Pyner, S., Booth, L., ... & Malpas, S. C. (2010). A novel low temperature transcutaneous energy transfer system suitable for high power implantable medical devices: performance and validation in sheep. *Artificial Organs, 34*(5), E160-E167.

4. Ranu, E., & MSBS, E. (2011). THE HIsToRy of scs dEVIcEs from fish to Electronics. *Essential Neuromodulation*, 213.

5. Liem, A. L. (2015). Modified from: How can spinal cord stimulation advance chronic pain treatment in 2015? Liem AL; Verrills P.; Bezemer R.; Almirdelfan K.; Levy R.; Kramer J. *Stimulation of the Dorsal Root Ganglion for the Treatment of Chronic Pain*, 165.

Made in the USA
Middletown, DE
23 August 2024

58994019R00130